A Woman's
Book of Life

A WOMAN'S BOOK OF LIFE

THE BIOLOGY, PSYCHOLOGY,
AND SPIRITUALITY OF THE
FEMININE LIFE CYCLE

JOAN BORYSENKO

RIVERHEAD BOOKS

NEW YORK

1996

Riverhead Books
a division of G. P. Putnam's Sons
Publishers Since 1838
200 Madison Avenue
New York, NY 10016

Library of Congress Cataloging-in-Publication Data

Borysenko, Joan.
A woman's book of life : the biology, psychology, and spirituality
of the feminine life cycle / Joan Borysenko.
p.   cm.
Includes bibliographical references and index.
ISBN 1-57322-043-4 (alk. paper)
1. Women.   2. Women—Psychology.   3. Life cycle, Human.
I. Title.
HQ1233.B76   1996
305.4—dc20   96-38374 CIP

Printed in the United States of America
9   10   8

This book is printed on acid-free paper. ♾

Book design by Chris Welch

I DEDICATE THIS BOOK,
WITH LOVE AND GRATITUDE,
TO THE MEMORY OF MY MOTHER,

LILLIAN FRANCES ZAKON,

AND TO MY DEAR FRIEND,

CELIA THAXTER HUBBARD,
AKA MOTHER GOOSE.

GOOD GOING, LADIES!

Author's Note

This book is based on life cycles common to all women, and issues that pertain to the majority of us. The special concerns of women of color, women who have emigrated from other cultures, disabled women, and lesbian women are important to us all, but were simply beyond the scope of my expertise. If any woman with special needs and concerns would like to share her experience, I invite you to write me at the address in the Resources section at the back of the book.

Acknowledgments

This book has been a labor of love, and its conception and birth, like all such events, has been collaborative. There are two people without whom this book would never have existed, and with whom I have had remarkable experiences of self-in-relation, a process through which something greater than either of us came into being. Mona Lisa Schulz, M.D., Ph.D., is a neuroscientist, psychiatrist, medical intuitive, and good friend. She did a substantial share of the research on which this book is based, as well as engaging me in some of the most stimulating discussions I have ever had. Her wit, enthusiasm, and prodigious intellect have enriched this book, and my life, tremendously. Amy Hertz, my editor at Riverhead Books, was invaluable in conceiving the idea for this project, and holding me steadfastly to its vision. Her remarkable insight, brilliance, clarity, and ability to see the forest for the trees have helped make this book what it is.

ACKNOWLEDGMENTS

· · ·

The ideas and experiences of many people, written and oral, have found their way into these pages. The groundbreaking work of Carol Gilligan, Ph.D., and her group at the Harvard School of Education; the late Grace Baruch, Ph.D., and Rosalind Barnett, Ph.D., of Wellesley College and their colleagues at the Stone Center, especially Janet Surrey, Ph.D., whose concept of self-in-relation is so central to female psychology; the late Yale psychologist Daniel Levinson, Ph.D.; Betty Friedan, who has brought us from *The Feminine Mystique* to *The Fountain of Age*; writer Gail Sheehy, who has taken us through many life passages including menopause; alternative physicians Christiane Northrup, M.D., who has put women's health and wisdom on the map, and John Lee, M.D., who has challenged the notion of menopause as an estrogen-deficiency disease, and "Era 3" physician and writer Larry Dossey, M.D., have been particularly important in guiding my thinking. Many other colleagues are mentioned in the text itself, or in the endnotes at the back of the book, and some are not. Herbalist Susan Weed, for example, is a wonder and I profited tremendously from her book *Menopausal Years* although her work is barely mentioned in the text. To any colleague whom I might have inadvertently omitted, you have my thanks and apologies. A book is rarely written by a single person, but represents a synthesis of wisdom arising from many sources.

Particular thanks go to Elizabeth Lawrence, M.A., my dear friend and partner in *A Gathering of Women* retreats, with whom I have shared so much, personally and professionally, in the last seven-year cycle of life. Thanks also to Jan Meier, M.P.A., our muse and musician at the retreats, and to Anne Disarcina, L.P.N., who sometimes joins us and adds her humor and wisdom. Thanks also to the women from the retreats who submitted their stories to me. Whether they were used in the text or not, they certainly added to my store of knowledge, touched my heart, and thus enriched the final project.

Some of the stories in this book were drawn from the years when I directed the Mind/Body Clinic at Boston's Beth Israel, and then New England Deaconess hospitals. To ensure the confidentiality of patients, all such stories are composites. While true to the processes that were demonstrated over and over again, none of them represents the life of any one individual, while embodying the spirit of many. Our fictional heroine, Julia, is also a composite of many women's stories, but largely a product of my imagination.

Special thanks to Robin Casarjian, M.A., Janet Quinn, R.N., Ph.D., and Christine Hibbard, Ph.D., who let me interview them. The interviews were so rich and moving that I wish I could have used more of them. Robin, who is director of the Lionheart Foundation Prison Project for Emotional Literacy, has been an incredible inspiration to social service and dedication to the spiritual life and a dear friend for many years. Janet helped sustain me with her outrageous sense of humor, great big heart, tremendous knowledge of healing, deep spiritual life, and fabulous friendship. Chris has been a real mainstay, a source of unending sustenance on every level. She cooked a lot of great meals, gave me journal articles, discussed the fine points of developmental theory, delighted me and my husband, Kurt, with her constant thoughtfulness, and has done the yeoman's task of reading several early, and cumbersome, drafts of this book. She's still talking to me, and that's a good friend.

Thanks to the Boulder women writers' group, good friends all, who held the vision for this book, bantered around ideas, and gave me critical early feedback on my first few tentative chapters. They liked it! Jan Shepherd, Judith Gass, Lynn Lundberg, Amina Knowland, and Janet Quinn, I cherish our friendship and look forward to many more shared creative projects. Even when I couldn't get to meetings because I was on retreat writing this book, your very existence was a comfort. Thanks to my other women friends whose wisdom and love have added so much. Peggy Taylor, Kristi Jorde, Ulla Reich-Henbest, Loretta LaRoche, Lynnclaire Dennis, Carolina Clarke, Carolyn Myss, Joan Drescher, Olivia Hoblitzelle, Beverly Feinberg-Moss, Rima Lurie, Rachel Naomi Remen, Eve Ilsen, and Celia Thaxter Hubbard, aka Mother Goose. Mentor and best buddy, I have no words to express my deep appreciation and gratitude for your love, Celia. Your bright mind, big heart, and nifty sense of humor are among life's greatest delights.

A special thanks to Judy Dawson, friend and administrative assistant, who was tireless in clipping articles and rounding up source materials that she thought I might find interesting. She also kept the world at bay, giving me the space I needed to complete the book, and made sure I kept getting to the airplanes on time so that I could continue with my primary work as a seminar leader, educator, and speaker. Judy, you're the best there is.

Finally, thanks to Looks With Wonder, aka Kurt Kaltreider, Ph.D., my husband. You are indeed the wind beneath my wings. Your commitment to the Native American culture of your ancestors, your tremendous base of knowledge in psychology, philosophy, and neuroscience, your willingness to cook lots of suppers, your help in rounding up books and articles, and especially your love have helped make this book a reality. Here's to the next thirty-seven years!

CONTENTS

CONTENTS

A Woman's
Book of Life

INTRODUCTION

THE FEMININE LIFE CYCLE

This is a book for women at every stage of the life cycle. It is not a primer for adjusting to aging, a treatise on how to bring our daughters through adolescence, or an attempt to prove that women have characteristics that make us superior to men. Instead, I have tried to present a rich and provocative understanding of the unique biology, psychology, and spirituality of women—a bio-psycho-spiritual feedback loop that confers specific gifts upon our gender that continue to unfold throughout the life span. As I've labored to bring this book into being, perhaps the most surprising revelation has been how little we women know of ourselves and how starved we are for information. Although this book is written primarily for women, I hope that it will be equally enlightening for men. For whether we are biologically male or female, each of us contains aspects of the other.

I recognize that to look for biological differences in behavior is sometimes to tread on dangerous ground. Geneticist Anne Fausto-

Sterling, in her fine treatise *Myths of Gender*, points out that at least in the field of brain research, scant differences have been found between men and women. We are far more alike than we are different, a fact reflected in the comment of Tufts University psychologist Zella Luria, who in commenting that overlap between males and females in most studies is greater than differences, said, "We are not two species; we are two sexes." And as many writers and researchers have pointed out, purported differences in biology have too often been used as ammunition to uphold traditional gender roles. With that caveat in mind, and with great respect for those who have labored to show how women's development, perceptions, and socialization differ from men's, I have decided to write this book specifically about women, rather than about male/female differences although I may occasionally refer to such distinctions to illustrate a point. Because the bio-psycho-spiritual feedback loop that determines femininity has not been explored previously, this book presents an entirely new vantage point for women's studies that I hope will be expanded on by many others in the years to come.

All human beings go through cycles in their lives, progressing from infant to child to adolescent to adult. While each stage builds upon previous biology and experience, evolving from one stage to the next sometimes requires a dying to what we have been in order to complete our metamorphosis. While the infant does not lament becoming the toddler, or the child mourn the approach of adolescence, women have been portrayed as lamenting our continued maturation into midlife and older adulthood. Older women are supposed to fade graciously— or gloomily—into the woodwork. Yet, as studies demonstrate, the truth is that women continue to develop their strengths and actually bloom, rather than fade, with the advent of midlife. Adolescent and young adult women, in contrast, experience much greater stress and insecurity.

Having asked more than ten thousand women who have attended lectures and seminars that I've given if anyone would like to be younger, I've had only one taker. Trading wisdom, experience, relationships—the pains and joys that create the fabric of growth—for youth seems an unattractive bargain, at least to some of us. While the groups of women that I've worked with are not a random sample of Americans, they are certainly the groundswell of a changing view about the nature of womanhood. The critical factor that unites these women is a deeply spiritual perspective that transcends differences in religious beliefs. From a spiritual vantage point our major life task is much larger than making money, finding a mate, having a career, raising children, looking beautiful, achieving psychological health, or defying aging, illness, and death. It is a recognition of the sacred in daily life—a deep gratitude for the wonders of the world and the delicate web of interconnectedness between people, nature and things—a recognition that true intimacy based on respect and love is the measure of a life well lived. This innate female spirituality underlies an often unspoken commitment to protect our world from the ravages of greed and violence.

While the aging woman may be grateful for the experience that has brought her wisdom, changes in her physical body may still be difficult to adjust to. The changes in my own midlife body at forty-nine, in fact, provided part of the incentive for this book. Every morning I greeted myself in the early winter light with the same ritual. Looking in the mirror with utmost seriousness I would pull the loose skin of my jowls behind my ears and contemplate the physical, emotional, and financial ramifications of a face-lift. I dealt with the loose skin of the lower regions of my anatomy by refusing to look in the mirror altogether. For two months I was sure that I was having hot flashes until I finally realized that they occurred only while I was standing under the bathroom lights for the protracted morning scrutiny. Even this was not reassuring, for I knew that menopause was surely on the way.

Despite my training as both a medical scientist and psychologist, I felt as confused about the coming changes as most of my friends. The only thing I felt for certain was that I was poised at the crest of a hill, about to take a big slide down into rapid aging and loss of sexual attractiveness. On the other hand, at forty-nine I also felt that I was just growing up, just becoming a woman. The Cherokees, in fact, believe that we don't enter adulthood until fifty-one. On my better days I had the exciting conviction that life was about to begin on a deeper, more passionate level than had been possible before. Two different voices were vying for control of my mind and emotions. The intuitive wisdom of the ages was calling for a celebration of rebirth into a deeper femininity. The societal myths about women and aging, on the other hand, were preparing me for the death of everything I had known and cherished about being female.

The need to understand the cycle of renewal in which I found myself led to researching women's evolving capacities. What are the beliefs that limit us and the wisdom that opens us up to greater possibilities? How does one cycle of our life prepare the way for the unfolding of subsequent seasons? How do the physiological changes we undergo in a monthly cycle during our reproductive years, and the continuing changes that occur after menopause, serve our evolution? What are the larger, cosmic cycles that entrain and lock us into these powerful rhythms? I began to notice the theme of seven-year cycles in sources as varied as the work of C. G. Jung, the Torah, the New Testament, the plays of Shakespeare, American folk wisdom, Native American tradition, Buddhist lore, the philosophy of the Greek mathematician Pythagoras, and naturally, in the phases of the moon that change every seventh day, and to which women's reproductive rhythms and hormonal pulses correspond.

Ancient Chinese philosophy, as described in *The Yellow Emperor's Classic of Internal Medicine*, employed a similar system of sevens for understanding how the structure of the female body parallels the workings of the universe. At seven, for example, a girl's secondary teeth come in and her hair grows longer. At fourteen menstruation begins and the girl becomes a woman capable of bearing children of her own. At twenty-one the woman is fully mature biologically and at her peak of function. At twenty-eight the muscles are described as firm, the body flourishing. At thirty-five, however, a cycle of decline begins. The face begins to wrinkle and the hair to thin. At forty-two the arteries begin to harden and the hair to turn white. At forty-nine menstruation ends and the woman can no longer bear children.

In ancient China men were portrayed as continuing to develop throughout the life cycle. As his body aged, a man grew in wisdom, morality, and judgment. Women, on the other hand, were not viewed as becoming wise—just as growing old and useless in a sexual sense. As a consequence they were devalued. Unfortunately, views aren't much different in twentieth-century America. When George Bush was elected president in his sixties, he was considered not only wise, but dashing and virile. First Lady Barbara Bush, on the other hand, was at first demeaned by the media as dumpy and old looking, a mean-spirited judgment that generated heated debate. Her body, a lovely example of older beauty, received much more attention than her bright mind and caring heart.

I have organized the female life cycle into twelve seven-year periods, three in each quadrant of life—childhood and adolescence, young adulthood, and midlife and the elder years. The thirteenth part of the life cycle, death, is perhaps the ultimate act of renewal and growth. Thirteen was originally the number sacred to women, corresponding to the number of months in the lunar year. Thirteen was eventually deemed "unlucky" because womanhood was considered a much less desirable alternative to manhood, an unlucky roll of the gender dice.

The female life cycle has traditionally been studied with reference to the three "blood mysteries"—menarche, childbirth, and menopause. These three physiological events mark the transitions between the three phases of life that have been recognized since ancient times—*maiden, mother, and crone.* This tripartite nature of the life cycle made sense physiologically until very recent times. In 1900 the average woman's life span was only 47.3 years. A leisurely walk through the graveyard in the historic old mining town of Gold Hill, Colorado, where I live, revealed a lot about that statistic. At the turn of the century, most of the graves were those of children. Often a whole family of young ones would die during a diphtheria or whooping cough outbreak. If a girl lived through the perilous passage of early childhood, childbirth was the biggest threat to her life as a young woman. Our little graveyard demonstrated that the few women who lived through childhood and childbirth often lived into their seventies, eighties, and nineties.

Women's life patterns have changed dramatically since the settlers moved to Gold Hill in the 1860s. By 1989 our expected average life span had increased to 75.3 years. Furthermore, if you live to be sixty-five, statistics predict that you can expect to live another 18.8 years—or until eighty-four. Because of the tremendous decrease in death from childhood disease and childbirth, there has been a monumental swell in the ranks of women in midlife, who are preparing to experience the third of the blood mysteries, menopause. Forty-three million women in the United States today are perimenopausal or postmenopausal and the number of women between forty-five and fifty-four will increase by one-half (from 13 to 19 million) by the year 2000. In contrast, the situation in developing countries like Pakistan is very similar to that in the United States a hundred years ago. Only 17 percent of the population is over forty. Middle age, then, is a relatively new phenomenon—at least in terms of the numbers of women in developed countries who have lived to this point.

Thus, the old concept of woman in her aspects of maiden, mother, and crone needs updating. The maiden years have gotten progressively shorter because electric lights and the subsequent elongation of the "daylight" hours stimulate the brain's pineal gland to release hormones that bring on puberty several years earlier, on average, than in the last century. We are also exposed to two sources of estrogen from external sources that have altered our natural hormonal balance: the estrogens used to fatten cattle and the "estrogen mimics" that are by-products of chlorine bleaching processes and pesticide manufacture. The latter, which are concentrated in animal fats and milk products, are called *xenoestrogens*, or "foreign estrogens," and are also probably related to premature puberty. Because of the earlier age of puberty, many mothers, are in fact, adolescents. For this reason, I have chosen to refer to the three seven-year cycles that extend from birth to age twenty-one simply as childhood and adolescence.

The mother years, too, have undergone enormous changes since women have had more freedom of choice about when, if, and how often they choose to mother. Physically and emotionally exhausted by a life spent pregnant, nursing, and caring for enormous broods, it was not unusual for women of previous generations to try to abort themselves and to die in the process, leaving their other children motherless. It was also common to die in childbirth of a ruptured womb that could not sustain the stress of one more delivery. And it was the rare wife who enjoyed sex since it was incontrovertibly linked to the terror of bearing yet another child. The family of today was unthinkable before birth control. We now take it for granted that if we are fortunate enough to be fertile and choose to parent, we can have the number of children that we can emotionally and financially care for. Unless divorce or the death of a spouse intervenes, we can then look forward to our midlife and older years in the company of our mates, children, and possibly our grandchildren. This happy family scenario was actually the exception rather than the rule before birth control. Since not all women of reproductive age mother, either by happenstance or by choice, I refer to the three seven-year cycles that comprise the years of twenty-one to forty-two not as the mother years, but as young adulthood.

When the potential mothering years are over, modern women enter the previously uncharted, unnamed midlife years, a time of life that used to be synonymous with old age. The modern woman in midlife is potentially wise, still vigorous, and in possession of a kind of fierce power that is biologically mediated by a relative increase in testosterone levels that occurs as estrogen levels diminish just before menopause. Ballsy behavior is supported by ballsy hormones. Tolerance for untruth, injustice, and disrespect for the rights of others becomes correspondingly low. A psychologically healthy midlife woman can be a serious challenge to dysfunctional families and institutions because of the tendency to be clear and vocal when the emperor has no clothes. I have chosen to name the midlife years the time of the *Guardian*—she who keeps the circle of life whole. The guardian is essentially a peace-keeper, but with the power to tell the truth and when necessary to be a warrior for justice. While the masculine aspect of the warrior is aggressive, the feminine aspect of the warrior is healing and transformative. After thousands of years of insanity—best defined as repeating the same behavior and expecting different results—it should be perfectly obvious that situations do not improve through violence and warfare. Rather, they are transformed through respect, relationship, understanding and love—the very qualities of the feminine that begin development in childhood and continue throughout the life span.

The crone, too, is a concept that desperately needs updating. In contrast to ancient Western perceptions of the crone as a snaggletoothed witch or the old Chinese perception that older women are useless and unattractive, the modern female elder is often a beautiful, savvy woman who uses the knowledge she has gained through the years, and the inherent spiritual wisdom of interrelatedness that continues to grow throughout the years, to impart values that support and encourage the growth of others and the preservation of life.

As we explore each seven-year period, we will consider the challenges that spur our growth during each cycle, the unique gift associated with each age, and some of the prejudices that have hindered women from expressing their full potential. For example, the inherent logical capabilities of women are discouraged when we are cast as emotionally more labile, more suggestible, and less analytical than men.

Women's differences have been seen as deviations from the norm, rather than as essentially different and worthwhile in their own right, in large part by taking men as the benchmark for human development. In fact, there has never been a theoretical framework for understanding women's development that wasn't based on a comparison to men. Even the most basic aspects of female anatomy are judged in relation to a masculine norm, as when Aristotle wrote that "Woman is an unfinished man, left standing on a lower step in the scale of development." Medical students learn the physiology of the seventy-kilogram man, and women are viewed as men with breasts, ovaries, and uteruses. This bias has led to a relative dearth of understanding of female physiology and many incidents that might be humorous were they not so pathetic. A woman asked her physician what effect a particular medication might have on her levels of estrogen and progesterone—the two most important hormones in determining a woman's cycles and the two hormones that make us different from men. The physician called the drug company that manufactured the medication and was assured that a study involving six hundred subjects had shown no effect on those hormones. Of course, the six hundred research subjects were men, and men don't produce estrogen or progesterone at nearly the level that women produce them. Psychological research has not fared much better. Until recently, almost all studies excluded women because menstrual cycling might produce mood or perceptual changes that would complicate the data.

Even career issues, and recipes for success in business adhere to a male viewpoint. Shortly after I joined the predominantly masculine world of academic medicine, for example, an older male colleague advised me on how best to get ahead. "Never show your belly," he warned, "or the sharks will move in for the kill." In other words, I should protect myself by showing no doubt, no emotion, and no vulnerability. This turned out to be an extremely isolating and defensive way to live. It gave me great compassion for men who have been socialized to fit such a mold. It also gave me a deeper understanding of the large body of medical literature that demonstrates how isolation creates stress that can lead to heart disease, immune dysfunction, and foreshortened life. Married male cigarette smokers, for example, have the same death rate as divorced nonsmokers. But if the smoking man is single, widowed, or divorced, his mortality rate doubles. Lonely people have a significant reduction in an important kind of lymphocyte called the natural killer cell that scours the body and eliminates cancer and virus-infected cells. Men who are widowed have a significant increase in illness and death for six months to two years after the death of their spouse. Women suffer no such ill effects upon being widowed, presumably because we have a much larger network of social connections than do men. Although the supposedly cardio-protective qualities of estrogen are usually cited as the reason why women live an average of seven years longer than men, it is likely that the social connectedness typical of women helps keep us healthier and confers longevity.

The prodigious research carried out over the past twenty-five years by women at Wellesley College's renowned Stone Center for Women's Research demonstrates that women are by nature relational, a trait that begins to develop in early childhood. While isolation is stressful for both men and women, it may be even more stressful for women since it is what psychologists call ego-dystonic. In other words it feels foreign, or dissonant, to our accustomed way of being. Eventually the stress of medical academia—of being a woman who was supposed to act like a man—was too much for me. In 1988 I defected from the Harvard Medical School and the Mind/Body Clinic that I had directed at one of the Harvard teaching hospitals for nearly a decade.

In the years since the "Great Defection" I've reflected deeply on how medical science and psychology have failed to consider women in our own right, rather than as men-in-the-making. As we progress through the life cycle considering women's development, I recognize that men may embody many of our same characteristics. My intent is not to elevate women above men, or to suggest that relationality and the spirituality of interconnectedness that grows naturally from our upbringing is strictly in the feminine domain. These are human traits that transcend gender. The physical, psychological, and spiritual development of men, however, is a rich and detailed field that needs little recapitulation here since it is the subject of volumes of work extending over many centuries. The corresponding book of women's lives is just beginning to be written. I offer this to you as a first, small chapter in that evolving work.

BECOMING A WOMAN

FROM ADAM'S RIB TO EVE'S
CHROMOSOMES

So the Lord God caused a deep sleep to fall upon the
man, and while he slept took one of his ribs and closed up
its place with flesh; and the rib which the Lord God had
taken from the man he made into a woman.
                                          —The Book of Genesis

One bright summer's day in the 1980s I was attending the wedding of friends who are conservative Christians. The marriage
homily started with the story of Eve's birth from Adam's rib and built
up to her legendary act of defiance. Eve, after all, was the temptress
who talked Adam into eating the forbidden fruit contrary to God's instructions. Therefore, stated the minister, a wife should listen to her
husband in all matters since women are inherently weak-minded and
easily tempted by evil. Nowhere in the telling of this old tale does anyone question Adam's judgment. After all, he didn't have to give in to
Eve and the serpent. He could have stood his ground and used his own
judgment. If we turned the tables on Adam and Eve, the parable could
just as easily be used as an example of male frailty.

Although some theologians argue that humankind *lost* free will because of Eve's disobedience, there can't be free will *until* a person can
consciously choose between what is life affirming and what is harmful.

In Eden, Adam and Eve had no choices, so they had no will. In one sense the biblical Paradise was a state of eternal early childhood without knowledge of the opposites that form the world. To their credit, both Adam and Eve chose to enter adulthood and accept the pain that is attendant to growth. To me, Eve is a metaphor for the highest level of women's bio-psycho-spiritual development. At the biological level she is a mother capable of bearing new life; at the psychological level she is willing to question authority and risk the unknown, even at the price of her own life, when her innate wisdom (the snake) suggests a way to enrich the world; at the spiritual level she appreciates that all things are related and interconnected, even the apparent opposites of good and evil. The preacher and I clearly had different viewpoints.

FROM ADAM'S RIB TO EVE'S CHROMOSOMES

Religion is not alone in elevating men while considering women morally, intellectually, and even physically inferior. The same frame of reference has pervaded science since its inception and persists subtly to this day in the types of questions that are asked both in the social sciences and in "hard sciences" like biology. The mystery of how eggs and sperm combine to yield males and females has been the source of endless speculation that only took a scientific turn in the 1950s when chromosomes could be reliably identified and the y-chromosome linked with male development.

Aristotle believed that "the male and female are related to each other as form and matter. The former is the active, the latter the passive part; the one bestows the motive and plastic force, the other supplies the material to be molded; the one gives the soul, the other the body." Women are simply raw material to Aristotle. The vital, intelligent molding force—and the soul—were associated with men, who were intellectually and spiritually granted higher ground.

And what determined gender to begin with? Aristotle believed that both men and women generated "procreative" substances. The menstrual blood of women was compared to "imperfect seed." It required the intelligent, organizing force of the male sperm to develop for "it alone [the sperm] contains the germ of sensitive life . . . the potentiality of the soul." If the male seed was warm and vigorous, Aristotle believed that a male child would be conceived. If the seed was cold and therefore less physically vital, a female would result. If the seed should be doubly defective—that is both cold and unable to imitate the paternal phenotype (external characteristics)—then the worst eventually would manifest. A girl resembling her mother would be born. It's little wonder, given the viewpoint of this well-known philosopher, that Western civilization has traditionally associated virility with the birth of sons.

The theories of gender development at the end of the 1800s were summarized in a British text entitled *The Evolution of Sex* which concluded that males were physiologically more evolved than women, who were nothing more than stunted men, a biological case of arrested development. Richarz, a leading theorist one hundred years ago, wrote that gender was determined by the "degree of organization" of the offspring. The healthier the mother and the more vital the offspring, the likelier it was to develop into the superior male. Were the mother weak, the resulting offspring would be less well organized, and thus female.

When I studied genetics at Bryn Mawr College in the 1960s, the molecular basis for gender differences had already come to light. In the early 1950s a researcher by the name of Jost discovered that the normal course of human development is female. He removed the fetal gonads (testes) from gestating male rabbit embryos and the resultant bunnies were normal females. He wrote that "In the absence of gonads, female development ensued. Therefore the development in mammals is in the female direction unless acted upon by some product made or regulated by the y-chromosome." I was exultant to discover that all embryos begin as females and only at the sixth week of gestation, under the influence of special antigens produced by the y-chromosome, do those destined to become male begin their differentiation. "Aha," I crowed to my mother on the telephone one day, "women don't come from Adam's rib—men come from Eve's chromosomes until their own get strong enough to kick in."

My exultation was short-lived. I soon began to hear these facts framed as a "default hypothesis." In other words, embryos were female by default, if they didn't have the special good fortune to inherit a y-chromosome. We were back to lack. The female lacks testosterone and is therefore deficient, an undeveloped male. This position went unchallenged for many years since it was completely in line with thinking that had extended back for millennia. Science often has a tendency to reflect the thinking of society, unfortunately, rather than to challenge it.

Very recently the old stereotype of women as biologically deficient men has been challenged and overcome. It turns out that women are not the default setting on the great cosmic biological computer. Instead, there are specific ovary-determining genes as essential for continuing female development as a y-chromosome is for the formation of male characteristics. In order for a male to develop, testis-determining genes on the y-chromosome must be activated to neutralize the ovary-determining genes. The default hypothesis also loses some of its luster when we look at some of the most basic interactions between egg and sperm. Mature eggs are different from any other cell in the body, engaging in incorporative and nurturing behavior. The ovum actively takes the sperm inside and supports the replication of its genetic material. Furthermore, eggs can repair sperm that are defective, including those with chemically induced mutations in the genetic code. In other words we appear to be programmed at a cellular level to fix the wounds of men—as my colleague Mona Lisa Schulz, M.D., Ph.D., quips—we are programmed to darn their physical, emotional, and even genetic socks!

The ovum also contributes genetic material to the offspring above and beyond what is present in nuclear chromosomes. A second source of maternal DNA resides in cellular organelles called mitochondria which provide energy for cellular reactions. Mitochondria are unique organelles because they are semiautonomous; they have their own genetic material (loops of DNA similar to those of bacteria) and reproduce by the simple act of self-replication. Without the necessity of combining their DNA with that of a mate, they double their own genetic material and then simply split in two, a type of reproduction known as binary fission used by bacteria and many other single-celled organisms. In fact, it is believed that mitochondria were originally bacteria that set up a symbiotic housekeeping agreement with human cells sometime near the beginning of our evolutionary history. We provided a home and they provided the complex energy-generating chemical reactions that allowed more complex cellular forms to evolve. The cells of one human being contain enough of these tiny, elliptical powerhouses so that if they were laid end to end they would encircle the earth twenty times.

While both egg and sperm have mitochondria, the egg is an enormous cell, while the sperm is little more than a nucleus with a tail that allows it to swim off in search of the egg. The few mitochondria that the sperm contains power its heroic journey, and are unceremoniously cast off when the egg incorporates the sperm's nucleus. The prodigious cytoplasm of the egg, however, is rich in mitochondria whose DNA helps direct nuclear genes and actively contributes to the development of the embryo. Cytoplasmic genes derived from mitochondrial DNA are thus contributed solely by the egg.

The fact that mitochondrial DNA comes only from the maternal line, and that these precious little symbiants are blessedly celibate (they reproduce all by themselves), has been exciting to anthropologists and biologists interested in the origin of the human species. The mitochondrial DNA in our cells today is very similar to what it was at the dawn of creation since it has not been contaminated by the messy genetic mixing that occurs when males and females pool their genes—since the sperm's mitochondria are lost when the egg incorporates the sperm. So in tracing the origins of mitochondrial DNA, biologists have also been able to trace our matrilineal family tree back to an African Eve, sometimes called Mitochondrial Eve, who lived somewhere between 150,000 and a quarter of a million years ago. Research teams led by biologists Douglas Wallace of Emory University and Allan Wilson at Berkeley sampled DNA from 135 women of diverse races—from Australian aboriginals to Europeans, Asians, Native Americans, Africans, and New Guinea highlanders. Even though the original mitochondrial DNA had naturally undergone some mutations during thousands of years of self-replication, a sophisticated computer search traced all women's common family tree back to a single Mitochondrial Eve. Researchers hasten to add two caveats: The existence of African Eve does not mean that all humans descended from a single woman residing in a biblical paradise—Eve was a member of a larger group whose members' lines of mitochondrial DNA simply died out along the way; and Homo sapiens is older than African Eve, suggesting that her lineage may have replaced more ancient populations.

The fact that there is an unbroken line of genetic information that has been passed from woman to woman through the ages, genetic information without which no embryo would develop, is final refutation of the old thesis that women are unfinished men. Without Eve's clever mitrochondria, and their ability to mend broken sperm and initiate embryogenesis, the entire human race would vanish. Perhaps an intuitive knowledge of this biological fact was responsible for the ancient custom of determining family lineage through the women. In the older "Goddess cultures," which were the norm until about five thousand years ago, all property was inherited through the women as was familial identity. Matrilineal descent is still followed in some cultures like Judaism. If the mother is Jewish, for example, the child is automatically considered Jewish no matter what the heritage of the father.

From this perspective, women are restored to their rightful place as partners in the evolution of humankind at the biological level. We become women not because we lack testes-determining genes, but because we have ovary-determining genes. And as women, our bodies have the capability of repairing damaged male genetic material to nurture the beginnings of a healthy new life. Now that we have put Adam's rib back in place and restored Eve's chromosomes to their rightful position, let's begin the journey of life by tracking the experience of a fertilized egg that, in the next chapter, will be born as a beautiful baby girl named Julia.

2

AGES 0–7:
EARLY CHILDHOOD

FROM EMPATHY
TO INTERDEPENDENCE

Julia is a composite woman whom we will look in on, from time to time, as she makes her way through the life cycle. Dealt a reasonably good genetic hand, and born into a hard-working and caring family, she was a full-term, healthy infant, the first child born to Sylvia, a bookkeeper in her late twenties, and John, a construction worker in his early thirties. Her only trouble was not uncommon. A fussy baby, Julia was colicky and hard to comfort, so her parents took turns walking around with her draped over a shoulder most nights. By the time Julia was three months old, their energy was wearing thin, especially Sylvia's. One night she just "lost it" and in a moment of uncharacteristic frustration and fury, she held Julia up as though she were about to shake her like a rag doll. Sylvia stopped herself—shaking a baby can kill it—and deposited Julia in her lace-trimmed crib, screamed at her, and then collapsed on the floor in tears. The baby was screeching in fear when John awakened, alerted by the ruckus. Fortunately for both mother and daughter, he was a patient, empathetic man. He gave Sylvia a hand up from the floor, took a moment to give her a hug, and then picked up his daughter and raised her above his head, looking into her eyes. "Hey, Princess," he crooned, "what's the matter?" Julia's furious cries gave way to big, throaty inhalations as he lowered her to his shoulder and began to pat her back, continuing to talk softly, unconsciously pacing the rhythm of his words and his footsteps to her quiet sobs. In a few minutes the sobbing gave way to deep breathing and Julia, thankfully no worse for the ordeal, slipped into a peaceful sleep.

Why are some babies, like Julia, easily aroused and cranky while others are placid? How does our response to their inborn personalities further shape their development? The answers to these questions lie in the intriguing area of neurobiology. But once the child's basic relationship to the world is in place at the ripe old age of eighteen months, are we likelier to respond differently to girls than we are to boys, creating persistent and identifiable patterns of female behavior?

NATURE AND NURTURE

Many children like Julia have nervous systems that are hyperaroused, on chronic overload. They respond poorly to strangers or new situations, like to sleep in their own beds, and can easily become snappish, irritable, and even inconsolable in response to common occurrences like waking up from a nap. These "difficult" babies are hard on their caretakers, who feel as though they should be able to comfort them, but often can't. Responses like Sylvia's are not uncommon, and when infants are shaken hard or repetitively, they can be seriously injured physically as well as psychologically when their need for comfort is met with anger. Fortunately for Julia, her mother was shocked by her own behavior, and the next time she reached a dangerous level of frustration, Sylvia counted back slowly from ten to one, calming down her own nervous system before it erupted in unconsidered fury. She was then able to respond to her daughter's needs more calmly, instinctually mirroring Julia's motions, verbalizations, facial expressions, and even breathing patterns just as John had on the night of Sylvia's emotional meltdown, and by six months of age, Julia's nervous system had begun to quiet down. Fortunately, our brains are wired in a way that allows emotional learning throughout the life span, as long as our caretakers are reasonably well attuned to our emotions and capable of mirroring them back to us in our first eighteen months of life. When caretakers are out of synch with the emotions of their child, however, she will fail to develop the empathetic connections that allow her to understand her own emotional needs in relation to those of others. She may become inherently narcissistic or self-centered, and relatively incapable of evaluating situations from other people's point of view. In the worst case sociopathy results, a condition in which other people are perceived as objects with no value other than to gratify one's own needs.

To understand how the most basic human attributes of empathy and emotional attunement develop, we'll begin with a brief foray into the exciting world of neurobiology where nature and nurture meet. While female brains do differ in some ways from those of males, the architectural wiring of this amazing three-pound organ is roughly the same in both sexes, producing hardware of nearly identical design. And a mutable hardware it is. The building blocks—neurons and a kind of connective tissue called glial cells—get lined up in their respective places, but only the basic survival circuits left over from our evolutionary days as reptiles and lower mammals get wired up according to an invariable plan. Much, but no one is sure just how much, of the remainder of the wiring—determining things like whether we get excited about Mozart or baseball; prefer to hike, write sonnets, get in fights, or plant a garden; whether we are rigid, demanding, and stress-prone, or calm, adaptable, and easygoing; whether we tend toward codependency or healthy interdependence—depends on how the basic components of the hardware get wired together by experience. Some of the circuits laid down in the first few years of life are metaphorically cast in stone. They don't change. But some of the wiring remains plastic and reprogrammable, which is why human beings can change, grow, and learn from our experience in ways that our distant ancestors, the lizards, cannot.

THE NEUROBIOLOGY OF EARLY CHILDHOOD

The brain begins to take form in utero as the outer (ectodermal) layer of the ball of embryonic cells called the blastocyst develops a little groove on its surface that deepens, fuses into a cylinder, and sinks into the rapidly developing embryo. The resulting neural tube multiplies at rates up to an incredible 250,000 cells per minute into a vast network of neurons that ultimately number in the vicinity of 100 billion. The neurons in turn sprout appendages that resemble long taproots, called axons, that carry electrochemical messages either to other nerve cells or muscles, and branchlike growths called dendrites that pick up signals from other neurons or from sensory organs like the eyes or ears. The little gap between a sensory organ and a dendrite, a dendrite and an axon, or an axon and a muscle fiber is called a synapse, across which an electric charge flows when neurotransmitters are released on one side of the synapse and picked up on the other. By adulthood the brain will have formed a staggering 100 trillion synaptic connections with exquisite sensitivity to signals from both the internal and external worlds.

Glial cells, which outnumber neurons ten to one, constitute much of the brain mass and perform a myriad of functions ranging from immune surveillance to cushioning the neurons like plastic foam pellets in a packing box. Glial cells also do a remarkable dance, wrapping their cell membranes around and around axons in concentric circles to create the myelin sheath, an insulating layer that improves electrical conductivity and makes circuits run faster and more reliably. The process of myelination is akin to transforming a twisting, rutted dirt road into a six-lane superhighway. The more a pathway is used in early childhood, the more it becomes myelinated, and the harder it is to change, which explains why our basic patterns of perceiving and responding to the world are in place by the time we are seven. If a little girl is repeatedly abused by a drunken father, for example, the resulting helplessness, rage, and fear of men are likely to be deeply embedded neurologically. Change is possible in later years by myelinating new pathways, but that change may require tremendous effort, considerable therapy, and sustained attention over many years since the initial circuitry will always remain.

When Julia was born, some of her neural pathways were already myelinated, hardwired into place. She could breathe, sweat, sleep and wake, turn her face to the side to find a nipple, swallow, digest, excrete, cry in protest, regulate her temperature, blood pressure, and heart rate. These mostly autonomic (automatic) functions are survival circuits. Unlike speech or intentional movement they occur without conscious will. In similar fashion, Julia was born with the ability to experience basic emotions linked to pleasure and pain, circuits that are likewise hardwired into place because they provide basic information about when our needs are being met and when they aren't, ensuring survival.

While teaching at Yale, neurobiologist Paul MacLean mapped what has become known as the triune, or three-part, brain. The oldest part of our brain, which looks like the stalk of a mushroom on which the rest of the brain sits, is responsible for instinctual responses and autonomic functions. Structurally, it is much the same as the brain of a reptile, whose rigid, obsessive, and ritualistic displays of dominance and submission lurk within us like a prehistoric throwback to earlier times. Perched atop the reptile brain is another holdover from furry cousins like cats and rats—the paleomammalian brain. Central to this second layer is the limbic system, a constellation of structures specialized for generating the emotions of pain and pleasure that are so critically linked to survival. If survival needs are thwarted, rage, fear, and pain result. When they are met, we experience pleasure. Unfortunately for irritable babies like Julia, the fear centers of her limbic system were too easily aroused, which, in turn, kindled similar unpleasant emotions in her mother. Neurobiologists often jokingly reduce limbic functions to the "four F's" of fighting, fleeing, feeding, and sex. From these basics, the more complex emotions of joy, rapture, grief, and empathy evolve with the appearance of the third level of the brain, the wrinkly layer of neocortex that gives the brain its walnutlike appearance and confers meaning on life's events.

Before we can generate meaning, our perceptual and motor functions have to mature, so that the first areas of the neocortex to myelinate are those responsible for sight, hearing, smell, taste, movement, and body sense. There are certain critical periods during development that are like transient windows of opportunity for neuronal hookup and myelination. For example, neurons of the visual system actively begin to sprout connections between two to four months of age and complete most of their basic wiring by about eight months. If a baby is born with cataracts that are not removed until the age of two, she will be blind for life. The window for visual wiring is closed. There are similar critical periods for learning phonemes or language patterns (the windows closes at about twelve months), and for becoming proficient at music. The latter window narrows considerably by ten years and is closely related to the circuits required for math and logic.

The window for empathy begins to narrow at about eighteen months of age when the newest evolutionary addition to the neocortex, the brain's massive frontal lobes which occupy the area in back of the forehead and account for 29 percent of brain mass, finish their basic hookup to the emotional limbic system. MacLean calls the frontal lobes the "heart" of the brain, waxing eloquent about the faculty of self-awareness and introspection that the frontal lobes provide, allowing us to develop relationships by identifying with the experience of other people empathetically through reading the emotion in their faces, putting ourselves in their place, and regulating our emotional response accordingly.

THE BASIS OF EMPATHETIC RELATIONSHIP

An attentive caretaker mirrors, or mimics, the behaviors, expressions, and vocalizations of a child. Julia smiles and her dad smiles. Julia pouts and Mommy pouts, matching her daughter's mood before she begins to pat her, bounce her, feed her, or sing to bring her child comfort. Julia waves bye-bye and her parents do, too. Seeing her own emotions and behaviors mirrored by loved ones myelinates the tracts between Julia's frontal lobes and limbic system. Then, when Daddy is sad, she perceives and mirrors his mood. She wants to comfort him as she has been comforted; she is empathetic. An infant who has been mirrored and comforted develops the ability to empathize even before she is aware of her own independent existence. In fact, newborn babies show a limited type of empathy by crying when they hear another infant in distress, a reflex called *motor mimicry*, which soon gives way to more active attempts to console others. When a friend's daughter, Jennifer, was about two and a half, for example, we were having lunch together at a restaurant. Jennifer was elbow deep in ketchup, methodically chomping her way through a plate of french fries. When I asked her for one she shook her head emphatically no and pulled the plate toward her protectively. I then pretended to cry, telling her that I was hungry. Jennifer's face instantly registered distress and she reached out a grimy little hand to comfort me, saying, "Don't cry. Jennifer feed you." Then she picked up a potato and put it in my mouth.

Relationship is the essence of life, and even newborn babies come wired to respond to human touch, speech, and facial patterning. Only hours after birth the infant moves her body in a precise synchrony with the speech patterns of her caretaker. By three or four months of age, human faces are a baby's favorite sight, and human voices her preferred sounds. By six or seven months even an initially cranky baby like Julia is likely to be disarmingly social, mimicking other people and hopefully being mimicked, or mirrored, in return.

The natural instinct on the part of a caretaker to respond to and imitate the baby through mirroring creates what psychiatrist Daniel Stern calls attunement—a playing back of the child's inner feelings. If these feelings are reinforced, the nerve tracts carrying them will sprout new axonal connections and myelinate. If not, they will weaken. So if baby Julia is joyful but her mother Sylvia is generally despondent, Julia will grow up relatively incapable of feeling joy. If Julia falls down and cries, she will develop empathy when Sylvia mimics her hurt, then picks her up and soothes her. But if Mother repeatedly yells at her for being clumsy, and fails to mirror other emotions as well, isolation replaces empathy and bonding is thwarted. In the most extreme cases, where children are left wet and hungry for hours or even days while parents are high on drugs, or when children in foundling homes are fed and changed on schedule, but not mirrored and responded to, they become physically stunted, prone to infection, and often die. The pituitary gland, which receives signals from the limbic system via the hypothalamus (which itself used to be called the master gland of the body), turns off the supply of growth hormone. If these children survive physically they do not thrive emotionally, because the circuits from the limbic system to the frontal lobes don't myelinate, and they can't form emotional attachments. Such children are likely to become sociopaths who feel no empathy for others and can rob, kill, and maim without conscience. Even when intervention begins at the age or six or seven, rehabilitation is a long and sometimes unsuccessful process because the empathy window has already closed.

BEYOND FREUD: EMPATHY, RELATIONALITY, AND INTERDEPENDENCE

If we are fortunate, like Julia, to have had a generally empathetic attunement with our caretakers, even though some instances of dissonance will inevitably occur, we complete what developmental theorist Erik Erikson called the stage of trust versus mistrust. If we learn to trust our caretakers, the developing cortex and limbic system wire in the basic belief system for an emotionally healthy worldview: "Life is a good gift and I can count on people meeting my needs." Whether we're female or male, this is the core belief that arises from the experience of an emotionally appropriate infancy.

As we enter the later childhood years, differences in the nurture of boys and girls begin to appear that shape our perceptions, interests, and use of the empathetic circuits that are already in place—valuable differences that are not generally appreciated in the male-oriented theories of development promulgated by Sigmund Freud and later by Erik Erikson. Freud, after all, believed that girls and boys not only develop differently, but that boys develop in a better way. His bottom line was not that men and women are different in interesting ways, but that women are inherently weaker-minded.

In order to construct a feminine view of the life cycle, we need to begin by sweeping Freud out of our collective unconscious closet. He might have had interesting insights about boys, but as far as girls go, penis envy is highly overrated. I can't help wondering if this theory was a projection of his own anxieties over the size of his male organ, an answer that unfortunately went to the grave with him. In any case, here's how Freud's theory unfolds. It is based on the Oedipus complex, a boy's innate longing to grow up, marry, and mate with Mommy, which Freud considered to be neurobiologically mediated. Boys are supposedly hardwired with this desire circuit. During the Oedipal phase, from three to five years of age, the little boy is in a nasty psychological bind since he begins to fear his father, who is a powerful, big and scary rival for Mommy's love. Unconsciously, the little boy fears the worst possible retaliation from his father—castration. Eventually this deep-seated and powerful fear helps the little boy push away from his mother, identify with his father, and develop the male characteristics of autonomy and independence that almost all life-cycle theorists have identified as the most important characteristics necessary for a healthy (albeit male) adulthood.

Resolution of the Oedipus complex is supposedly what makes men independent, autonomous, and manly rather than dependent on Mother like the inherently weaker little girl who is lacking a penis and cannot act out the same intrapsychic drama to push away from her mother and achieve independence. The ability to live in isolation—almost as though other people don't exist—is touted as a prized male quality. Furthermore, we girls are supposed to spend our childhoods feeling inferior to boys, wondering what could have happened to our prized male part. This supposedly sets the stage for a life of relatively low self-esteem and failure to differentiate into autonomous, interesting people. Rather, we are said to live on psychically connected to our mothers, in a continually dependent position.

Female developmental theorists like psychologists Nancy Chodorow and Carol Gilligan, whose book *In a Different Voice* is a classic, have rightly pointed out that autonomy and independence are indeed intrinsic to male development, but that little girls develop a different, and just as important, quality, that of relationality. Rather than having to repress maternal characteristics like empathy and tenderness to differentiate from Mother, little girls adopt these qualities. Affiliation and relatedness become the ground out of which a healthy sense of self grows—not in distinction to others, but as part of a worldview in which relationship is the crucible in which autonomy, creativity, compassion, and wisdom are forged. The women researchers at Wellesley College's Stone Center have worked together through ongoing colloquia to define a concept of women's sense of self in relation to others that is a model for the inherently feminine view of life as an interdependent web of mutually enhancing relationships. Psychologist Janet Surrey of the Stone Center writes that "Our conception of the self-in-relation involves the recognition that, for women, the primary experience of self is relational, that is, the self is organized and developed in the context of important relationships." The prized quality here is to live in the realistic context of the existence of other people. Male development, in contrast, is predicated on separation from the mother and the continuing development of a sense of autonomy—a sense of self-in-isolation rather than a self-in-relation.

What is meant by self-in-relation? We don't exist any other way. We exist in the context of other people, other beings and environments. The key concept is one of interdependence, an understanding that relationship provides a context in which all participants can grow and become empowered, the emergent whole evolving into more than the sum of its parts. That we can become greater beings through relationship of any kind is, I believe, the very soul of the feminine worldview. When the three-year-old Julia smiles at her mother and thanks her for helping her take a bath, if Sylvia is really open to receiving her daughter's gratitude, her heart opens and her self-esteem is enhanced. Something emergent, greater than either Julia or Sylvia, comes into being and the relationship takes on a spiritual quality.

Janet Surrey further distinguishes healthy relationship from attachment. The latter term implies that the other person is an object of gratification whereas relationship implies the ability to identify the relationship as an entity larger than one's own self, coupled with the intention to nurture and care for that evolving entity. Western culture socializes little girls along relational lines, whereas little boys are socialized in accordance with a competitive, autonomous model. When children's modes of play are analyzed, little girls tend to play in smaller groups than do boys, engage in less competitive games, and relate more cooperatively.

Research suggests that the relative ease with which girls attune to others is also a function of differences in the ways that girls and boys are taught to deal with emotions. Psychologist Daniel Goleman cites data that parents are more prone to discuss emotions (other than anger, which is presumed to be unladylike and therefore more likely to be denied or glossed over) with their daughters than with their sons, show more emotions when playing with female infants, and use more emotion words with girls than with boys. Little Julia is therefore more likely to be able to tell her parents that she is sad, joyful, peaceful, lonely, afraid, confident, or loving than a little boy of the same age. Since girls learn language skills before boys do, "this leads them to be more experienced at articulating their feelings and more skilled than boys at using words to explore and substitute for emotional reactions such as physical fights. . . ."

THE GENDER CONTROVERSY: EMPATHY AND SUBORDINATION

The recognition of relationality as a female developmental trait has stirred the boiling pot of gender controversy. Some commentators like Susan Faludi, author of the popular book *Backlash*, see relationality as a throwback to the kind of soft, weak stereotype used as fuel for the belief that women are best kept barefoot and pregnant, functioning as kinkeepers and supports for more powerful men who get the "real" stuff done. Researcher Carol Tavris makes the additional point that while women have long been judged by the yardstick of men, it is equally critical not to judge men by the yardstick of women or to ascribe differences to either gender that do not exist. For example, in *The Mismeasure of Women*, she cites evidence that because many people subscribe to the notion that women are more empathetic than men, when psychologists ask research subjects to rate their empathetic skills, women generally rank higher than men. However, when studies are performed that measure physiological response to the suffering of another, men and women score equally. Both sexes also respond equally in terms of behavior—doing something to alleviate another's distress—although women in daily life do seem better able to "read" other people's emotions and behaviors than do men. Interestingly, this talent may turn out to be more of a survival skill than a gender difference. In experiments done in pairs, when one person is in charge and the other is subordinate, the individual of lower status quickly learns to attend to the nonverbal cues of the "boss" no matter what their gender.

Empathy, Tavris suggests, may be more of a power issue than a gender issue. Although many people subscribe to the notion that women are no longer subordinate to men in our culture, that perception is currently at odds with the way in which little girls in Western culture learn about society. At the most basic level, the message a child gets from watching television is that women are sex objects whose power is derived from pleasing men whereas men are powerful in their own right including their ability to be violent and exploit others through robbery, war, and rape.

The fact remains that in most cultures, little girls are raised in a milieu in which men have been accorded the power, and are therefore socialized in the subordinate position. Neurobiologist Jerre Levy, doing brain lateralization research at the University of Chicago in the 1970s, discovered that the female right cerebral hemisphere has different functions than the male right hemisphere. It is less specialized for making sense of spatial relations and more attuned to emotion and the understanding of facial expression. If Sylvia is sad, for example, and she doesn't want to acknowledge her feeling verbally, it is still likely to show on her face. Little Julia, because of her ability to read facial expression, may be more likely than her father to notice her mother's feelings and to mirror them. Put another way, John is more likely to make the logical assumption that since Julia is acting cheerfully, she is cheerful even if her face tells another story. He will therefore relate to her differently than Julia will. The little girl's ability to go beyond what is said to what is felt confers the ability for what the Stone Center group calls "relationship authenticity," the "ongoing challenge to feel emotionally 'real,' connected, vital, clear, and purposeful in relationship." While this relationship skill may be a result of the societal subordination of little girls, it still exists by virtue of differences in the overall socialization of girls and boys.

THE CONFUSION OF RELATIONALITY WITH WEAKNESS

The idea that relationality is a weakness, and autonomy a strength, can be related back to a more feminine-centered look at the work of Erik Erikson. During the ages from two to five, when Freud zeros in on the Oedipal conflict, Erikson focuses on the resolution of a developmental crisis that he frames as initiative versus guilt. If Julia is consistently mirrored and acknowledged for climbing trees, solving problems, or striking up conversations with strangers, for example, she is likely to learn initiative. But if she is shamed for being bold or outgoing, she is more likely to learn that these behaviors are unacceptable, and thereby end up as a helpless, guilt-prone adult.

The young child is a great explorer and adventurer. I am often delighted in supermarkets and airports (where I spend a lot of time) with little children who spontaneously strike up conversations, ham it up looking for an audience, climb up on trash cans and grin as they balance on their perch, sing songs at the top of their voice, offer cookies to strangers, or race around creating games. The responses of their parents are interesting to observe. Sometimes a child is scolded or physically pulled away. The parent may be embarrassed that the child is disturbing someone, irritated at having to chase her, or fearful that the child will be hurt or abducted. At other times the parent may join the conversation or in some other way encourage the child's act of socialization and initiative. Since little girls are particularly adept at reading the nuances of emotions on people's faces and in their tones of voice, they can easily learn that adventurous behavior causes, fear, anger, or guilt in their parents. Exploring and performing behaviors may be seen as unladylike or potentially dangerous. Little Roger, for example, is more likely to be encouraged or simply humored for playing hide-and-seek by crawling under the feet of a stranger in an airport gate area than is Julia. And if we are scolded and shamed for being adventurous, the lesson is likely to be a lasting one. I want to emphasize the point here that little Julia is inherently no less autonomous and adventurous than Roger. Because she has been socialized to be more responsive to the emotions of others, she is more easily shamed and prone to lose her initiative to explore and perform because of guilt that she has made her parents feel bad.

When children feel shame they show obvious physiological signs of helplessness and submission like blushing, shallow breathing, burying the head, or averting the eyes. This behavior is wired instinctually into the reptilian and paleomammalian brain (the limbic system). Humans are pack animals, and when the head dog shows disapproval to an upstart lower in the hierarchy, the underdog puts his tail between his legs, lowers his head, and slinks away. This behavior keeps the peace and calls off potential attack by the alpha male. The emotion that accompanies this neurological circuit in humans is called shame.

Psychologists have referred to shame as the "master emotion." It is so uncomfortable and isolating that one wishes to avoid experiencing it again. Therefore, anatomical pathways are laid down so that we will remember the shameful situation and be better equipped to avoid it. Those pathways run between the limbic system and forebrain, eventually constituting the "executive functions" of morality—the software that reminds us of what's right and wrong, socially acceptable and unacceptable. Shame is intrinsically an "isolating" emotion since it accompanies incidents in which we have displeased the "tribe," which might then abandon us. The potential for abandonment, which to our paleomammalian brain is equivalent to death, mobilizes a potent fear response. The adrenaline surge that accompanies fear activates the vagus nerve, which regulates heart rate; the vagus also relays messages to the amygdala, an almond-shaped structure within the limbic system that imprints emotionally intense memories. Julia only needs to be shamed for taking the initiative to talk to strangers a handful of times before she will begin to avoid it. The fear of loss of relationship is a particularly powerful negative reinforcer.

Girls who are repeatedly shamed for taking initiative are likely to grow up helpless. Helpless people believe that they are incompetent to bring about change in the world and in their lives and are likely to be passive, pessimistic, prone to depression, and to develop a host of psychosomatic ills. They are easily stressed and less able than others to come up with innovative solutions and ideas. This set of behaviors may look like a lack of autonomy and independence, but it is actually an emotional consequence of the shame circuit. My own mother was a study in helplessness and the fear that attends it. Every time I climbed a tree, talked to a stranger, or ran ahead on a walk I was shamed for making my mother feel afraid. She was so concerned that something might happen to me that she lay in wait outside the bathroom door, calling anxiously if she thought I was inside too long. In addition to chronic constipation due to lack of privacy, the result was an enduring case of self-doubt that might have been far more serious if my father hadn't encouraged my curiosity and initiative. Nonetheless, for many years I had a tendency to second-guess my decisions. Were they right? Might I inadvertently hurt someone? Was I causing someone discomfort?

Helplessness, guilt, and pessimism are obvious blocks both to the expression of healthy relationality and to autonomy. Ironically, attempts to keep little girls safe and train us to be ladylike can result in a deeply ingrained pattern of self-doubt that inhibits our ability to act. As mothers, aunts, friends, and grandmothers charged with the care of a new generation of women, we might reflect on Gertrude Stein's words, "Considering how dangerous everything is, nothing is really very frightening." Within reason little girls need the freedom to explore, to exult, to climb trees, and to become themselves. Yes, there are dangers lurking out there, but perhaps the greatest danger overall is the failure to nurture courage and initiative in our daughters. Without that nurturance, we will raise another generation reflecting the myth of the helpless woman.

BEYOND RELATIONALITY TO THE RATIONALITY OF INTERDEPENDENCE

I was driving along in a companionable silence with a niece of mine when she was about six. She turned to me suddenly with a beatific smile on her face and announced cryptically that words were wonderful things because they contained information about many worlds and how the different worlds touch. When pressed for an explanation, she said that a tree had to do with the world of the sky—the sun, rain, and wind. It also had to do with the earth and the worms. Everything was connected. Little Alexa had stumbled upon the concept of interdependence.

Alexa had grasped the reality that nothing exists independently of anything else. This is in stark contrast to the way our culture thinks of objects as intrinsically different and isolated from other objects. When we think of a simple word like *cookie*, we often don't pay attention to the fact that its existence is dependent on the growth of a wheat field and the micro-organisms that live in the soil. The soil is filled with the richness of ancient flora and fauna, which lived and died eons ago, leaving their skeletons as a legacy for future generations. The cycles of darkness and light that sustain photosynthesis, the climatic variations that produce wind and rain, the force of gravity, the exact distance of our planet from the sun, and innumerable evolutionary forces are necessary to grow wheat, sugar cane, and cocoa beans for the cookie. Then

consider the labor of the countless people who are involved in producing a single package of Oreos. The farmer's very existence is dependent
on his parents, whose existence is dependent upon countless ancestors.
Then there are those who harvest the wheat, pack it, ship it, truck it,
mill it, sell it, buy the flour, bake the cookies, run the factory, balance
the books, truck the cookies, stock them in the store, sell them at the
counter, give them to the child, and gain or lose from investing in the
company's stock. Perhaps the master baker and his wife make love one
night, and his resultant state of relaxation is so profound that he drifts
into a particularly sound, sweet sleep and has a creative dream that
leads to improvements in the recipe. Cutting down the rain forest
changes the climate, which in turn affects the wheat. Nutrients in the
wheat sustain life, while a caffeinelike substance in the chocolate shifts
the body energy of the consumers. Little Paul offers Julia a cookie,
which causes her, in turn, to smile at the postman who was having a
bad day but now feels better. Pesticides in the wheat accumulate in the
fat of those who eat the cookies, leading to breast and prostate cancer,
and a reduction in men's sperm counts. Some are born, others die, and
the molecules of a simple confection are part of it all. All these interdependent worlds in a single cookie, and we've barely scratched the
surface. When my six-year-old niece brought up the word "tree," this is
the reality she was beginning to understand. This is the reality of the
feminine development of self-in-relation, the reality that often puts
women at the forefront of movements to save the environment and
movements to improve conditions for children.

Most female developmental theorists have discussed relationality,
but have stopped short of the inherent logic that extends the understanding of self-in-relation to others to self-in-relation to all that is.
When we take time to think of the logical ramifications of interdependence, it becomes clear that nothing exists in isolation. Every act,
thought, and deed is like throwing a stone in a pond, creating ripples
that are theoretically infinite. This point of view is inherently logical,
feminine, and an obvious extension of the view of self-in-relation.

My belief is that all children who make it through Erikson's stage of
initiative versus guilt, and continue to develop empathy, possess the intrinsic neurobiological pathways that can evolve into Alexa's understanding of interdependence. Because females in our culture are
socialized relationally, they will naturally be more prone to continue

developing circuits that support an understanding of interdependence in their early childhood. The socialization of boys toward autonomy and independence, however, may interfere with similar development, which may therefore take longer to emerge.

Many indigenous cultures socialize both genders in ways that lead to an inherent understanding of interdependence. Most Native American and aboriginal cultures, for example, base their lives on the understanding that everything is interrelated and that what we do today has to be extrapolated seven generations into the future. The concept of nurture and respect for life doesn't have to be taught, because it is a natural spiritual consequence of how their children are raised.

THE INNATE SPIRITUALITY OF CHILDHOOD

Young children often have a kind of natural wisdom, a mindful appreciation of the present moment, that is instinctual. They sometimes perceive things that adults do not, like angels and imaginary playmates. Excursions into fantasy may be encouraged for little girls more than for little boys. The educator Rudolf Steiner believed that children live in a kind of dream state until they reach the age of seven. This dream state, which may involve the same kind of expanded view of reality experienced in indigenous cultures, may correspond to the fact that the right hemisphere of the brain matures before the left. Until about seven thinking is intuitive and holistic, what psychiatrists and developmental theorists often call "magical thinking." Rocks and cars, dolls and stuffed animals are perceived as conscious, living entities—a form of animism that persists in some of us as adults. Do you ever find yourself talking to your car when it won't start?

Freud called the right-hemispheric type of perception that underlies the childhood dream state *primary process*. Although Western cognitive theorists generally malign primary process as a developmentally primitive mode of cognition (thinking), it bears a striking resemblance to the way in which many wise indigenous peoples view the world. Consider the Australian Dreamtime, for example. In the aboriginal Creation myth, Baiame (the creator) lay sleeping. He dreamed earth life as it was in times past, present, and future. Baiame got so excited in the dream state that he began to shake, thus awakening three spirit helpers from another dimension. The three beings offered to help him materialize his dream. From the Supreme Intelligence that was Baiame, they took tiny portions called *yowies* (souls). These souls could then manifest the dream of earth through their ability to mold form from thought. The earth and plant worlds were created, but the sun goddess, Yhi, had to be called on to create the right conditions to nurture higher forms of life. She, in turn, called on Ularu, the Intelligent Snake from the spirit realm. A great rainbow appeared and that wise being known as the Rainbow Serpent slithered down and burrowed out the earth to create seas and mountains. Souls who had been minerals and plants could now create the animal kingdom and continue to dream evolution into creation.

The sun goddess and her snake helper are one of many ancient myths that informed the later Creation myth of Genesis. In the Old Testament, however, Eve and her snake have been demoted to cosmic miscreants. The primary-process thinking characteristic of Dreamtime has likewise been demoted from the inherent wisdom of childhood to primitive, childish thinking.

We might infer from studies of hemispheric myelination that intuition (our connection with the Dreamtime) develops before the capacity for language, since the right brain myelinates before the left. Since little girls are encouraged to "play make-believe" more than little boys are, the right brain in girls has a greater richness of development that underlies the ability to read emotions from facial expressions and the perception of self-in-relation. These same right-brain pathways are involved in intuitive, holistic thinking, the perception of the dreamtime.

It is said that the Creation myth of the Dreamtime was given to the aborigines about ten thousand years ago at a time of crisis and famine, that they might remember their connection to spirit and learn to function in a new environment. In a fascinating account of aboriginal history, Cyril Havecker writes, "He [Baiame] sent a message by clear sentience and because every animal, plant, mineral and human has a portion of the Great Spirit's Intelligence, and were at the time, highly developed psychically, they were able to receive the Great Spirit's message with ease."

Children up to the age of about seven are similarly developed psychically, although evidence for their life in the Dreamtime may be missed because it is devalued. The standard schemes of childhood development all stress cognitive skills and are oriented toward exiting the dream state. As a result, ways in which babies and small children communicate other than through language or symbolic gestures are virtually unexplored. My very first memory was of lying in a baby carriage outside the apartment house where we lived. My mother had stopped to talk to another mother, also wheeling her baby in a carriage. I was not only aware of the communication between the two mothers, which I understood perfectly, but was also communicating with the other baby.

As childhood progresses, and we begin to develop language skills, the left hemisphere myelinates. This probably correlates with the development of the linear, rational thinking that emerges in middle childhood, after the age of seven. Some children of both sexes retain intuitive skills, even as logical thinking develops. In general, however, primary-process skills are more easily accessed by women than by men because of the fact that the right hemispheric pathways through which women become especially attuned to reading emotions, and developing the skills of self-in-relation, are also involved in intuitive perception.

The bio-psycho-spiritual basis of the feminine life cycle is wired firmly into place by the end of early childhood, conferring the gifts of empathy, relationality, interdependent perception and intuition. These gifts have the potential to continue their development, becoming amplified both through experience and continuing biological changes, through the remainder of the life cycle. When they are recognized and encouraged for the remarkable strengths they are, the feedback loop that sustains these gifts is amplified and the virtues of compassion and interrelatedness that they support naturally unfold in our personal and collective lives.

AGES 7–14:
MIDDLE CHILDHOOD

THE LOGIC OF THE HEART

Our friend Julia, now seven years old, is at Thanksgiving dinner at her grandmother's house. Her parents, four-year-old brother, Alex, and about twenty other members of the extended family just finished an enormous meal and have settled down in smaller groups to have coffee and chat or to watch the football game. Julia, her mother, Sylvia, Aunt Anne, and Grandma Sharon curl up on a window seat under a New England-style leaded glass bay window that overlooks a little stream, its banks heaped with an array of multicolored leaves. Sylvia crosses her legs, leans forward, and begins, somewhat proudly, to discuss John's promotion to senior job supervisor at the construction company where he works. Julia pipes up, "Yeah, and it's a good thing that he got the job, too, or we would have had to sell our house because the payments were so much. There were too many bills and he was mad at Mommy for spending so much on clothes. They are kissing more now," she concludes, "and that makes me feel better."

In three sentences, Julia has summarized her family's financial and emotional situation. Sylvia wasn't even aware that Julia knew about these matters, and doesn't know whether to laugh or reprimand her daughter for telling the family secrets. She settles for a middle ground, complimenting Julia for her insight, agreeing that everyone feels much better now, and explaining that these are very personal matters that are best kept within the family. Julia counters, with perfect logic, that Grandma Sharon and Aunt Anne *are* their family. The art of facade has not yet begun to develop and total honesty is the order of the day.

Girls in middle childhood are extremely perceptive about relationships and feelings, and also feel free to express themselves, often to the embarrassment of their parents. This natural ease makes middle childhood a charmed period for children like Julia who have been encouraged and cared for by emotionally healthy parents. Heidi and Pippi Longstocking come to mind as literary archetypes of the exuberant energy and relational charms of middle childhood. In comparison to boys, studies show that girls of this age are more resilient and optimistic, verbal, articulate, and sociable. Harvard psychologist and researcher Carol Gilligan, whose interview studies of young girls and adolescents have charted new territory in women's development, observes that young girls naturally comment on relationships, note violations of trust and intimacy, and feel compelled to tell the truth even if they get in trouble for it.

TOWARD A LOGIC OF MIND AND HEART

While interactions like Julia's Thanksgiving Day proclamation are typical for little girls, who have already mastered the logic of the heart, they are far less frequent for male children. But at about this time, new psychoneurobiological circuits mature that give both genders the ability to use linear, sequential, mathematical logic—a stage of development at which little boys initially excel. According to the well-known theories of developmental psychologist Jean Piaget, we shift into a more adult mode of thinking, called the period of *concrete operations*, at about the age of seven. The primary developmental test for this emergent stage of logic is called *the law of conservation* which can be demonstrated with a simple test. If two beakers of the same size are filled with water, children under seven can say that they are equal. But if water from one beaker is poured, for example, into a tall, thin container the young child is likely to think that it holds more water than the shorter beaker. Once having reached the stage of concrete operations, however, the child knows that the two beakers hold the same amount even though one looks as if it holds more.

The left-hemispheric function that matures during middle childhood confers the ability to sequence and serialize, to understand part-whole relationships, and to make classifications. It is not, however, a more *advanced* form of logic than the early right-brain thinking that forms the basis for perceiving the kinds of subtle interconnections between people, events, and emotions that young Julia demonstrated when she commented on how her parents' worry about money was affecting their moods and their relationship, and how the entire picture shifted when her father got his promotion. Both kinds of logic are important and necessary, even though most psychological theories continue to tout the importance of linear logic circuits while denigrating the importance of the earlier logic circuits of the heart that support the perception of relationality—if you'll recall the example of the cookie and my niece's perception about the tree.

In this chapter we'll explore the ways in which girls in middle childhood develop the capacity to use linear logic while retaining the interrelational, interdependent perceptual capability they developed in early childhood. When these two sets of circuits function together, the left-brain logic of concrete operations complements the right-brain logic of primary process and a refined, penetrating kind of perception results. Once again, I am not implying that boys can't form and conserve the same circuits, only that differences in socialization may selectively strengthen the use of both circuits in girls.

Recent neurological data does, in fact, suggest that women are more likely to use both kinds of pathways than are men. Neurologist Bennett Shaywitz and his wife, pediatrician Sally Shaywitz, headed a research team at the Yale Medical School that used functional magnetic resonance imaging (a brain-mapping technique that detects very small changes in blood flow indicative of brain activity) to investigate the way in which the nervous system converts letters on a page into sounds. Although they were not looking for male/female differences, fascinating data emerged in the area of rhyming. Picking out rhymes caused an increase in blood flow to Broca's area (the inferior frontal gyrus of the left hemisphere which has long been known to relate to language ability) in both men and women. But in the majority of women (eleven out of nineteen), the corresponding area of the right hemisphere was also involved. We can infer that the eleven women who represented rhymes on both sides of their brain were able to conserve more "developmentally primitive" right-brain pathways while simultaneously adding the left-brain pathways that Piaget was concerned with in cognitive development. This two-track level of perception may also be involved in the recurring debate about boy/girl differences in moral reasoning during middle childhood.

THE HEART LOGIC OF MORAL DEVELOPMENT

At eleven, Julia came home from school one day with a shocking announcement. The parents of her best friend, Gwen, were getting divorced. When she asked her friend why, Gwen responded that her father had fallen in love with another woman because her mother acted mean a lot and made her father feel bad. Gwen felt bad for everyone. She was sorry for her mother and wondered what her father's role might have been in causing the meanness that he had cited as a reason for falling in love with another woman. She was also angry at her father because she thought that adultery was a betrayal of the whole family. She was sorry for her brother and herself, as well as "the other woman," whom she felt she would never learn to love and would therefore always feel like an outsider. Julia looked at how all the different worlds touched each other. Her twelve-year-old brother, Oliver, however, had a different take on things. As mean as his mother might have been, adultery was worse than yelling and his father had to shoulder the entire blame for the divorce. Oliver was furious at his dad, and refused to speak to him at all.

Julia was full of questions at the dinner table that night. Was it better for parents who were unhappy to stay together for the sake of the children? Was adultery a worse sin than meanness? Would marriage counseling help? Could Gwen and Oliver ever form a decent relationship with their stepmother-to-be when they thought of her as wrecking their family? And what of poor Oliver? It would be hard enough to weather his parents' divorce without being estranged from the father that he now said he hated with all his guts. What was right and what was wrong?

The question of whether boys and girls differ in moral reasoning has been hotly debated. Carol Gilligan's premise in her 1982 best-seller, *In a Different Voice*, is that they do. Other research strongly suggests that gender plays no role in moral decision making. In reviewing these data, I have concluded that researchers are often comparing apples and oranges. Both girls and boys are capable of making moral decisions, they just get there using different types of logic.

Let's start by reviewing the steps of cognitive development that lead up to moral decision making. As middle childhood progresses, according to Erik Erikson, the preadolescent ideally masters feelings of inferiority through suitable industry that leads to the production of tangible results. At eleven, Julia enjoys a wide range of arts and crafts. An avid reader, she also writes stories about the adventures of Aaron the Aardvark, with which she entertains her little brother, Alex. The child now knows enough of the workings of the world, the "rules of the game," that she has reached a state of autonomy in which she can think things through for herself and solve the problems of the adult world logically. Julia, for example, understands that adultery is a betrayal; it is wrong. During middle childhood, pathways in the prefrontal lobes have been myelinating, creating well-worn pathways that confer the capacity for moral comparisons based on what the child has come to deem socially acceptable or not acceptable. According to Piaget's scheme of cognitive development, the child of about eleven has entered the stage of *formal operations*, a level of thinking epitomized by "reversibility thinking." This is the capacity to consider a problem from numerous points of view, all potentially valid, and then return to the starting point. Formal operations presupposes that we have developed a stable point of reference, a framework for thought, to which we return after assessing a situation's possibilities. Julia's starting point in thinking about Gwen's parents' divorce is that adultery is wrong. But like Gwen, she then considers the possible mitigating factors, and the nuances of relationship and behavior that have led to the betrayal. Piaget linked cognitive development to how we make moral judgments. But as you will see, his system encompasses linear logic and male thinking brilliantly, but does not extend to the female tendency to use the right-brain interrelational intelligence of the heart in tandem with left-brain, linear logic.

During early childhood, Piaget described a stage called *moral realism* in which rules are seen as sacred, permanent, and unbendable. Since thinking at this time is primarily egocentric, a child cannot fathom that other people may operate from a different point of reference or that situations may arise that necessitate changing the rules. When Julia was four or five, for example, she saw the movie *Robin Hood* and deduced that the hero was a villain because he stole things. The possibility that stealing from the rich to give to the poor might be morally acceptable, righting a previous wrong, did not exist in her black-and-white thinking. This type of rigid God-will-get-you-for-it point of view is characteristic of fanatics and dogmatists.

During middle childhood, between the ages of seven and ten, we ideally enter the stage of *moral independence*, a more flexible point of view in which rules can be modified if necessary. There is a world of difference between these two stages. To the young child, the amount of damage done when a mistake is made is much more important than one's intentions. A five-year-old Julia may cry inconsolably over spilled milk. A ten-year-old Julia doesn't get so upset because the damage was unintentional. And ten-year-old Julia now sees Robin Hood as a hero. Assessing the *motivation* for an action becomes of primary importance.

Psychologist Lawrence Kohlberg extended and modified Piaget's theories of moral development into six stages. Some people, as you will note from the following description, never reach the more advanced levels. In stages one and two (*the preconventional level*), judgment of right and wrong is egocentric and hinges on what you have to lose or gain personally. In stages three and four (*the conventional level*), judgment falls in line with societal values and laws. In stages five and six (*the postconventional level*) judgment is tied to a set of ethical values that may supercede societal laws.

In *In a Different Voice*, Carol Gilligan contrasts the answers given by a boy and girl of eleven on a standard test of Kohlberg's moral development. The two sixth-graders, whom she calls Jake and Amy, were equally bright yet their answers seemed to confirm Kohlberg's findings that "the edge girls have on moral development during the early school years gives way at puberty with the ascendance of formal logical thought in boys." The children were presented with a moral dilemma in which a man named Heinz cannot afford to buy a very expensive drug necessary to save his wife's life. The pharmacist refuses to lower the price. The question is, should Heinz steal the drug? What is more important, life or property? Jake is very clear that Heinz should steal the drug, and when he is interviewed he can give a clear and logical set of reasons that uphold his opinion. Furthermore, he is delighted with the problem—he compares it to solving a math puzzle whose steps are obvious.

Amy's answer is far less assured. She wonders about other solutions since neither stealing the drug nor letting Heinz's wife die seems reasonable. For instance, perhaps Heinz can borrow the money. Amy's interview does not serve to clarify her position. There are so many variables, all of them seen in terms of relationship. How many people would be hurt by the death of Heinz's wife; how might the druggist feel if his failure to respond results in her death; what about the relationship of Heinz to the druggist? Gilligan sums up Amy's responses, "Failing to see the dilemma as a self-contained problem in moral logic, she does not discern the internal structure of its resolution; as she constructs the problem differently herself, Kohlberg's conception completely evades her . . . seeing a world comprised of relationships rather than of people standing alone, a world that coheres through human connection rather than through a system of rules, she finds the puzzle in the dilemma to lie in the failure of the druggist to respond to the wife."

According to Kohlberg's system, Amy's moral development is inferior to that of Jake. The problem, according to Gilligan, is that Jake and Amy are trying to solve different problems. His is a problem of logic, hers of human relationship. While Gilligan's premise was widely hailed throughout the 1980s, gender differences in moral reasoning using Kohlberg's scales have not always been borne out and a number of theorists have tried to counter her arguments. Men and women seem more alike than different in moral reasoning—and yet the vignette of Jake and Amy rings true for most of the men and women that I've described it to. The logic of most studies, however, is typically male and bottom line. Were the scores equivalent or not?

A completely different question, and the one that Gilligan was really addressing, is how do boys and girls *reach* their conclusions—

whether or not their conclusions are comparable? She wanted to know why, if women reasoned in a different way from men, it was considered inferior or problematic. Journalist Susan Faludi criticized Gilligan's research and her emphasis on the different logical/moral pathways that girls use on the basis that to be labeled "different" in our society is tantamount to being pigeonholed as handicapped. Furthermore, she maintains, when girls are portrayed as primarily relational, antifeminists can turn this idea into a backlash by stating that independence is therefore an "unnatural and unhealthy state for women," and that we are thus unsuited for the work world and should remain at home as nurturers.

Perhaps we could move this tired debate to another level, out of the sphere of independence versus relationality and into the sphere of interdependence—the recognition that we are all related on a variety of levels, from the societal, ecological, political, and spiritual to the atomic. Another way of viewing the dilemma of Heinz, for example, is that its very existence is a moral failure of Western civilization's overreliance on the mind logic of isolation and lack of appreciation for the heart logic of interdependence—a social feature that adversely affects both males and females. Isolation affects immune function as well as psychological development. How could we ever have reached a point where the cost of a drug could be measured against a life? If we persist in solving problems from the point of view that Jake took, which supposes that events are isolated rather than connected, we will continue to create similar moral dilemmas. How, in a supposedly "advanced" society, for example, can we weigh the life of one person against another based on their ability to afford health insurance or to qualify for Medicare or Medicaid? How can we think that cutting down virgin forests to create jobs in the short run could fail to initiate a chain of ecological disaster that will affect many generations to come?

The Dalai Lama speaks eloquently about the synergism of heart and mind—and the crucial distinction between independence and interdependence as we mature. He writes, ". . . when we get older, we sometimes feel we are completely independent; we don't need others' help, and we ourselves are everything. We neglect the positive value of affection. . . . Though the knowledge of our brain is developing, the other human quality—the good heart—is not catching up. Because of this, knowledge becomes more destructive, more negative. Today the world is very complicated, and much suffering has happened due to lack of human sympathy and human affection. . . . If the whole planet suffers, we will also suffer. If the whole planet gets more peace, more harmony, we will get the same. Therefore each individual has a responsibility for humanity."

The Dalai Lama's moral reasoning is quite similar to Amy's, emphasizing the interdependence through which every action creates consequences whose ripples extend through many levels, ultimately coming back to ourselves. This type of logic is an innately spiritual feedback loop that arises from and helps to cultivate a compassionate heart. The idea that independence often fosters a neglect of the positive value of affection is crucial. If we isolate ourselves from one another, failing to develop an affectionate, emotionally mature self-in-relation through which both parties evolve greater wisdom and compassion, linear logic and its unfortunate consequences will continue to prevail as the dominant system of Western morality and behavior. Expanding on Kohlberg's six levels of morality, I would suggest that interdependent reasoning is a seventh level, a spiritually based morality, that Amy so aptly demonstrated.

BRAIN, MIND, AND INTERDEPENDENCE

The gift of interdependent perception accompanying the myelination of pathways between the limbic system and the frontal lobes that occurs during early childhood is augmented by the continuing myelination of the frontal lobes during middle childhood. While the "heart of the brain" continues to develop, morality becomes a hardwired affair as the beliefs that give meaning to our life become biological pathways. The nature of interdependent perception, however, also involves other areas of the brain, most important of which is the right temporal lobe of the neocortex, located, as its name implies, beneath the right temple. This part of the brain has been dubbed the "circuit board for mysticism," since stimulation of this area gives rise to a direct perception of interdependence, the sine qua non of spiritual experience. Furthermore, as we will discuss in this section, interdependent thinking may involve an aspect of mind and perception unrelated to the brain entirely.

Dr. Wilder Penfield was a neurosurgeon who worked at the Montreal Neurological Institute during the 1940s and 1950s. When neurosurgery is performed the patient is given only local anesthesia for two reasons: the brain doesn't feel pain and while talking to and observing the patient the neurosurgeon can electrically stimulate the region of the brain slated for removal to make sure that the memories of a patient's family or her ability to use her legs are not being sacrificed by mistake. Penfield made remarkable progress mapping the different motor and sensory areas of the neocortex while performing such surgeries. Some of the most interesting of his discoveries involved the brain's temporal lobes.

When the brain was stimulated in the region of the Sylvian fissure, an area of the temporal lobe above the right ear, patients reported out-of-body experiences, hearing celestial music, talking to God or dead relatives, having experiences of interdependent perception where everything seemed connected with everything else, and even having a life review. These kinds of observations have led some scientists like astronomer Carl Sagan to the position that near-death experiences (NDEs) and mystical states are simply by-products of the firing of temporal lobe pathways with no objective reality. In other words, the brain is a computer made of meat and all subjective mystical experience can be reduced to the firing of neurons. Penfield, too, compared the brain to a biological computer, but he fervently believed that the mind was not an emergent property of neurons, the output of a machine, but an enlivening principle—the energy and blueprint that allowed the computer to run in the first place. Is it possible to choose sides in such a debate?

Many people who have had an NDE (and according to a Gallup poll, that's one person in twenty in the United States) subjectively experience that their mind is outside of their body. Dozens of patients that I've interviewed over the years have reported floating through hospital walls and observing surgeries and other events elsewhere in the building, wishing to see their families one last time and finding themselves observing the action in the family living room, or accompanying paramedics on their trip from the dispatch area to the scene of their own resuscitation. But anecdotes do not science make. Cardiologist Michael Sabom decided to devise a test of whether patients were really outside their bodies or just imagining the experience. He interviewed a random sample of patients who had been clinically dead, most from cardiac arrest, and were subsequently resuscitated. Forty percent of those patients reported an NDE with some combination of the classic components consisting of having an out-of-body experience, moving through a tunnel, experiencing extraordinary peace and love, seeing dead friends and relatives, meeting a transcendant being of light, and reviewing one's life. He interviewed thirty-two patients who had been brought back from cardiac arrest to ascertain whether they could actually report details of their resuscitation that they could only have known if their mind was hovering over their body during the procedure. These patients recalled surprisingly specific details of their resuscitation, described the sequence of events with uncanny accuracy and even reported the conversations of the team. The clincher was that some NDE-ers reported visual details that would only have been apparent if they were, indeed, looking down from the ceiling rather than picking up impressions through some unconscious mechanism while lying flat on a gurney. Furthermore, when twenty cardiac patients who had not had NDEs were asked to describe the resuscitation procedure, they made numerous mistakes.

So, does the brain have a mind that is greater than the sum of its synapses? We might use the analogy of the brain as a television whose wiring allows it selectively to pick up multiple signals that are traveling through the air, but can only be decoded and perceived when they are received by the set. Although the machine's wiring is critical to the production of picture and sound, no matter how carefully the television is dissected into its component parts, we will never find the little man inside (the mind) who is reading the news. Some neurobiologists, like mystics, have concluded that the brain exists within a unified field of informational vibration, the mind, rather than the mind existing within the brain. Our thoughts and behaviors seem to interact with and change this vibrational field. British biologist Rupert Sheldrake, for example, has hypothesized that unified fields of information, or morphic fields, are capable of producing alterations in the physical world. When psychologists first began to send rats through mazes, it required a longer period of time for a "naive" (untrained) rat to learn the maze than it did several years later. It is as though the cumulative experience of the rats created a field of intelligence which other rats could tap into, a kind of "hundredth rat" effect.

Do these data, and the involvement of the right temporal lobe in the direct perception of interdependence, have a particular relevance to women? My hypothesis is that they may, although specific research would be needed to confirm my hunch. Psychologist and researcher Kenneth Ring at the University of Connecticut has gathered the most comprehensive database available on NDEs. Of 111 persons whom he included in his first comprehensive study, 80 people—72 percent of his sample—were women. He hypothesized that the preponderance of women was due to the fact that women were more likely to write to him and describe their experiences than were men. There is, however, an alternate hypothesis. Since only about one in four people who are judged clinically dead actually report an NDE, perhaps women are more likely to recall the experience than are men because of some base-line differences in temporal lobe wiring that might make it easier for them to retrieve such experiences in the normal waking state. People with dissociative disorders in which normal daydreaming proceeds to a vivid sense of distancing from the body and engaging in other activities, and people with multiple personality disorder (MPD), often display unusual capabilities reminiscent of temporal lobe activation including feelings of leaving their bodies and traveling to distant locations. The majority of people treated for these conditions are also women. Psychiatrist Frank Putnam, an expert on dissociative states, reports that the female-to-male ratio of MPD cases is approximately five to one.

One of the most striking features of NDEs has to do with relationality and interdependence, modes of thinking that we have also traced to female development. One of the most fascinating commonalities in NDE reports is that the experiencer perceives everything as being connected to everything else and comes to believe that every thought and action affects everything else. One of my patients for example, who "died" as a result of a severe allergic reaction to penicillin, reported that her life review consisted of vignettes of relationships she had had. The most surprising thing for her was that she could see how her interaction with others affected their subsequent interactions with others ad infinitum, as in a hall of mirrors. Once again, the concept of isolation and interdependence is highlighted. When people report life reviews, rather than reviewing the relationship from an independent perspective, they experience interactions as if they were in the body and emotional state of the other person.

Interdependence also has correlates in the fascinating world of quantum physics. When quantum theory began to be explored with Einstein's 1905 discovery of the theory of relativity, a whole field of "strange" and "spooky" physical phenomena began to mystify scientists. Bell's theorem, for example, states that once two atoms have been part of a molecule and then separated, no matter how far distant they are from one another, each atom acts as if it is still in communication with the other. Since the atoms that make up molecules are forever trading places, it is quite possible that right now you may have atoms in your body that once belonged to Mother Teresa, Adolf Hitler, your mother-in-law, and even Sigmund Freud. Furthermore, these atoms remain interconnected with all other atoms that they have ever been related to. These kinds of phenomena led Albert Einstein to observe that the perception that we are separate from one another is an optical delusion of consciousness, about as clear a statement of interdependence as can be made.

The right temporal lobe may be the neurological circuit for transcendant experiences of interdependence. People with temporal-lobe epilepsy (often referred to as complex partial seizures) in fact, are often preoccupied with religious thinking and may feel compelled to write volumes about their relationship to the universe. They may report out-of-body experiences and also frequently report strange feelings akin to electrical discharges that originate at the base of the spine, give rise to orgasmic flows of energy, can cause their body to contort into yogalike postures, and sometimes lead to insightful revelations.

This "body energy," which is unexplored and unnamed in Western science, forms the basis of medicine in many other cultures, like China, where the energy that enlivens the body is called *chi*. In fact, forty-nine different cultures have a name for this enlivening force that is believed to run through the body in specific channels, known in Chinese medicine as *meridians*. Blocks in the flow of *chi* can be relieved by certain types of massage, acupuncture, emotional adjustments, time spent in nature, certain combinations of herbs, and a variety of meditation practices known collectively as *internal chi gong*, or work with body energy. Furthermore, the energy can be passed to others, a form of healing known as *external chi gong*. *Chi* is a good analogy to what Wilder Penfield called mind, the enlivening force of the body and brain. The growing field of complementary medicine takes such energy into account, suggesting that the more technical approach of Western allopathic medicine (the "body-as-machine" approach) can be improved by simultaneously using methods that stimulate the body's innate healing mechanisms, or *chi* flow, and taking into account the interdependence of each patient with the natural world, the emotions of other people, and her relationship to the cosmos.

The question about interdependence that intrigues me most is not its existence, but how it has been forgotten in Western culture, allowing the ascendance of a linear logic that is critically important, but not as primary to morality and to the preservation of life for future generations. It may seem logical to develop nuclear power, for example, but what of the problems it may create later, problems adequately demonstrated by the nuclear catastrophe at Chernobyl that has poisoned soil in many European countries, so that crops cannot be grown because they contain too much radioactivity for human or animal consumption? The myth that women are too emotional and not logical enough can be cast in a very different light by considering the logic of the heart. The perception of interdependence and interrelatedness is, in fact, an elevated form of logical thinking that informs an intrinsic morality and spirituality that is more associated with female than male development in Western culture. The onset of puberty, for women, presents another developmental impetus in this direction, but menstruation, like so many other aspects of female psychophysiology, has been cast in a negative light.

REINVENTING PUBERTY

My bunkmates and I were juniors at Camp Pembroke in Massachusetts where I spent every summer between the ages of eight and fifteen. It was a languid August afternoon, and we had about half an hour between swimming and volleyball to change our clothes and rest. A few friends and I were just settling in for a game of jacks when ten-year-old Vicki began to scream. These were not the screams of a girl who had fallen and hurt herself, or even the screams of a girl who was afraid of spiders, which Vicki was. They were screams of abject terror. One of our counselors went running into the bathroom where the commotion was centered. Vicki had just become the first of us to get her period, and at ten years old was entirely unprepared for the experience.

I remember feeling both sorry for Vicki and envious at the same time. Vicki was a woman now, capable of bearing children. She had passed through some magical portal and although she still looked like a child, she was not. It seemed awesome and mysterious—but why was she so frightened? I wondered if there was something about getting one's period that I didn't know, something much scarier than what my mother and the fifth-grade grapevine had passed along. But rather than talk to Vicki, or to the counselors, most of us talked amongst ourselves, isolating our friend because we were afraid of what had happened to her. Some of us knew the basic biological facts about menstruation thanks to a pamphlet that the Kotex Company published in the 1950s. We were also convinced that getting your period hurt, was bad smelling, messy, embarrassing, itchy, and uncomfortable. Many of our mothers called it "The Curse."

Earlier that year my mother had fumbled through a rudimentary discussion of the birds and the bees. It ran something like this. "Soon you will get your period, which is described in this booklet." She handed me the famous Kotex Manifesto. "It's a terrible inconvenience, as you know," (I had walked in on her in the bathroom often enough that I knew The Curse involved a lot of bleeding, pads, and toilet paper) "but you'll get used to it. The main thing is," she lowered her voice ominously at this point, "after you get your period you can get pregnant. And boys are only interested in one thing. Sex. And you're the one who'll have to pay the price. If you get *pregnant*," she fairly hissed these sinister words, "you will *ruin* your whole life and *disgrace* the family. No *nice* boy will *ever* want to marry you. So *never*, absolutely, *never*," (I remember her agitated finger pointing at about this place in the lecture) "let a boy take advantage of you" she finished with a weak innuendo, "if you know what I mean."

I did know what she meant, sort of. We girls had discussed the ins and outs of the sex act if you'll pardon the pun, spicing up what we didn't know with what we could conjure up. In our giggly, wide-eyed imaginations boys got some kind of period, too—a time each month when they manufactured those trillions of tiny sperm—and this was the only time that a girl could get pregnant. Compared to today's ten-year-olds we were woefully ignorant. At eleven, our friend Julia was hiking a mountain trail with her mother, Sylvia, and her aunt Anne. Julia was already experiencing some of the wondrous changes that culminate in puberty. Her breasts were budding and her hips were already those of a woman. Anne and Julia struck up a conversation about the miraculous metamorphosis that Julia's body was undergoing. Smiling and laughing with an easy camaraderie, they compared notes about such exciting events as finding hairs in one's armpits. Julia told Anne about an absolutely wonderful program she had seen on public television that had really helped prepare her for what was happening. Her knowledge was precise, coupled with great excitement and a sense of reverence for the mystery of entering womanhood.

Jungian analyst Judith Dirk, in her powerful book, *A Circle of Stones,* asks of puberty and other rites of passage, "How would it have been different if?" Have you ever wondered about this? How would it be different if our mothers gave us a sense of excitement and mystery about being a woman, if getting one's period was not coupled with the fear of pregnancy, if we knew that our dreams and our entire reality were about to undergo a major shift, if we thought this passage a blessing rather than a curse?

The notion that menstruation is a curse, a punishment for Eve's sins and a sign of the degenerate nature of woman is an ancient belief. Pliny the Elder, a Roman naturalist who was a contemporary of Jesus, summed up the thinking of the time when he wrote that a menstruating woman will "dim the brightness of mirrors, blunt the edge of steel and take away the polish from ivory." As late as the sixteenth century, medical authorities promulgated the myth that demons were produced from menstrual blood. According to a Persian tradition that predated Christianity, the first woman was seduced by a serpent and immediately began to menstruate—a belief echoed by Jewish rabbis, who thought that the curse of menstruation was a result of Eve's dalliance with the snake in the Garden. The poor maligned snake, however, was once the symbol of wisdom and regeneration rather than a sign of death and the devil, as the Australian Dreamtime myth of the Rainbow Serpent who helped the sun goddess create the world reminds us.

In indigenous cultures including those of Native Americans, menstruation is viewed as a time of positive power, rather than as evidence of sin and negative power, or as a feminine inconvenience. Menstruating women are segregated from the tribe and prohibited from taking part in ceremonies not because they are "dirty," but because they are thought to have an expanded connection with universal energy at this time which is so powerful that it could effectively short-circuit a ceremony or affect the energy bodies of other people. Jamie Sams, a Seneca medicine woman, states that a woman's "moontime" is a particularly propitious moment to connect with the Orenda—the spiritual essence within each person that is connected to the Great Mystery. Failure to do so, she strongly believes, may contribute to illness and burnout, another reason why women traditionally repaired to the moonhut so that they could use the natural opening that menstruation provided to rest and commune with a larger reality.

The Mohave Indians place great significance on the dreams that occur during menarche. Young girls are instructed to remember all their dreams, which are then shared with a wise elder of the tribe. The girl's future life can then be predicted and guided on the basis of information that she has retrieved from the dreamtime—our connection to an expanded, interdependent reality. C. G. Jung similarly discussed puberty as a time of awakening to states of inner knowing that may sometimes be confused with psychotic states, as in the case of the "voices" that instructed the adolescent Joan of Arc, who some theorists believe might have suffered from right temporal lobe seizures.

THE ANATOMY OF PUBERTY

Is there, in fact, anything about the physiology of menstruation that might support the belief that puberty provides an expanded opening to greater power and knowing, or an attunement to extracorporeal energy? At puberty an adolescent woman's body does become minutely attuned to lunar energy cycles. Studies have shown that peak conception rates (and thus ovulation) occur at the full moon or the day before, and that maternity wards are also noticeably more crowded when the moon is full. During the new moon, ovulation and conception rates are decreased overall, and an increased number of women start their menstrual bleeding. The lunar cyclicity of the menses is orchestrated through the interlocking effects of four hormones: follicular stimulating hormone (FSH), luteinizing hormone (LH), estrogen, and progesterone. To understand how these hormones interact, we need to consider four separate organs: the pineal and pituitary glands within the brain, the ovaries, and the uterus.

The *pituitary* gland responds to myriad subtle influences including emotions, stress levels, sex, nutrition, pheromones, the sight and smell of one's beloved, and day length. The pituitary, in turn, is acted on by another gland buried deep within the brain, the *pineal*, which secretes the neurohormone *melatonin*. The pineal, filled with little crystals called brain sand, is actually a vestigial third eye whose capacity to respond to changes in light/dark cycles regulates both the circadian rhythms of the body and tells the pituitary when it is time to begin secreting the hormones of puberty. In other animals, most notably birds, it orchestrates time of birth to coincide with the season in which the young are most likely to survive. The French philosopher René Descartes called it the seat of the soul. And perhaps it is, since many cultures believe that the onset of menstruation is associated with a profound awakening of power, intuition, and a capacity to access knowledge from other realms. In Eastern cultures, the pineal corresponds with the sixth chakra, or third eye. So perhaps at puberty, when the output of hormones from the pineal is at its peak, we have a literal opening of that wisdom eye.

In the days before electric lighting, the mean age of puberty for girls was fourteen or fifteen. Artificial light, plus a diet high in fat, which contains both the estrogens used to fatten animals and estrogen-mimicking chemicals derived from organochlorine-based pesticides and by-products of paper whitening called dioxins, have affected modern girls so that the mean age of puberty is now between eleven and twelve. When the pineal signals the pituitary that the time is right, the latter gland begins to produce FSH and LH, and the young woman's entire body begins to respond to cycles of moonlight as well as sunlight. Under the influence of FSH, several ovarian follicles—little sacs of cells containing an undeveloped egg—begin to ripen in the time between menstruation and ovulation. This is called the *follicular phase* of the cycle. The cells of the follicles themselves mature and produce several types of estrogen, the predominant variety being estradiol, while the egg grows in size. At ovulation, one, or occasionally several, eggs are released.

Following the release of the egg, the follicular cells that remain behind are transformed into a temporary endocrine (hormone producing) organ called the *corpus luteum* which means "yellow body." The corpus luteum manufactures progesterone, which, in turn, causes the lining of the uterus to thicken and become ready for a fertilized egg to implant. During the so-called *luteal phase* of the cycle, the endometrial inner layer of the uterus becomes rich in glycogen, a storage form of sugar. Blood vessels actively proliferate and interpenetrate the uterine lining cells, preparing to bring nourishment to the fertilized egg that may implant there. If pregnancy does not occur the corpus luteum functions for only ten to twelve days, producing both estrogen and progesterone. When it closes down and progesterone levels fall, the lining of the uterus is shed as the menstrual flow.

Do the hormonal changes that occur during the cycle affect women's perceptual abilities or emotional lives? A study done by a psychoanalyst, Dr. Therese Benedek, and physician, Boris Rubenstein, in 1939 is often cited in this regard. The two worked in different cities. Benedek kept notes on the women's emotional and dream lives, while Rubenstein looked at slides prepared from their vaginal mucous, a technique through which the phase of the menstrual cycle can be documented. In the follicular phase, when estrogen levels were high, women were outgoing and creative. In the luteal phase, when progesterone levels were high, they were more inner directed. During ovulation women were content and receptive to being cared for, research that has been more recently confirmed.

Gynecologist Christiane Northrup has expanded on the reports of Benedek and Rubenstein. She compares the premenstrual and menstrual phases of the cycle to the dark of the moon. "Women, too, go through a period of darkness each month, when the life-force may seem to disappear for a while (premenstrual and menstrual phase). This is natural. We need not be afraid or think we are sick if our energies and moods naturally ebb for a few days each month. . . . Studies have shown that most women begin their menstrual periods during the dark of the moon (new moon) and begin bleeding between four and six A.M.—the darkest part of the day.

PMS AS A POSITIVE BIO-PSYCHO-SPIRITUAL FEEDBACK LOOP

What if the need to be alone, to be still, to stare at the wall, that many women report during their time of moon dark is not a dreadful disease called premenstrual syndrome (PMS)? What if it is the body's natural call to tune in and reflect, opening ourselves to greater wisdom? Jungian analyst Ann Ulanov describes the feminine consciousness as periodic and rhythmic. We wax and wane. "At ovulation," she says, "a woman's body is receptive and fertile. She may then feel an emotional expansiveness, an abundance of sexual energy, a new potency in her creative ideas and inspirations. If her ego is not in touch with this phase of her cycle, she often squanders her energy in increased busyness."

On the basis of clinical observations in her practice, Dr. Northrup believes that if we routinely stay busy and block the natural flow of information that comes to us in the luteal, premenstrual, and menstrual phases of the cycle, then we are more likely to experience symptoms of PMS. Both Dr. Northrup and I have observed that women tend to become preoccupied with negative ruminations in the latter part of the cycle. Things that may be bothering us, but that we are unwilling to confront, tend to come to light as if they are being flushed from the unconscious to the conscious so that we can attend to them. Perhaps, for example, fourteen-year-old Julia is concerned that her steady boyfriend is two-timing her, but she wants to believe that it isn't so. Denying her feelings and hunches, she tries to carry on as usual. Her stress level mounts, and just before menstruation, her hunches break through in the form of disturbing dreams in which her boyfriend makes fun of her or takes another girl to the freshman dance. During the day she feels nervous and irritable as she tries to keep her mounting tension under wraps. Her adrenaline and cortisol (an adrenal hormone that increases when we experience chronic stress), begin to rise. The adrenaline makes her jittery and anxious. The cortisol, which is an anabolic or tissue-building hormone, makes her hungry. She binges on sugary snacks that, in turn, make her lethargic. She craves salt, which makes her retain water, and begins to feel miserable, which she attributes to the coming of The Curse. If she were willing to discuss her mounting fears of infidelity with her boyfriend, she might find that her symptoms were a blessing in disguise, leading to the resolution of an emotionally difficult situation.

I was in high school during the infamous Cuban missile crisis and while politics have never been my strong point, I do remember an interesting debate that arose during that time. Was a woman physiologically suited to be president? The argument went something like this. Of course not. What if she had PMS when trouble erupted in a place like the Bay of Pigs? One confused, bitchy woman—driven by a powerful hormonal storm—could unleash the nukes and bring the world to an end. This line of reasoning, which sought to bar women from positions of political authority in the 1960s, was no different from an argument made by the Philadelphia County Medical Society over a hundred years earlier when they attempted to bar women from medical training with the argument that our cyclic changes rendered us weak, confused, and constitutionally unfit to deal with crises in the practice of medicine.

Brown University geneticist Anne Fausto-Sterling suggests that these derogatory perceptions of premenstrual "craziness" may have infiltrated medical views of PMS. In particular, she calls the work of Dr. Katherina Dalton, the British physician who coined the term *PMS*, into question. Dalton made headlines through such extreme gestures as testifying in the trial of a woman who purposely killed her boyfriend by running over him with her car. Because she suffered the temporary insanity of PMS, suggested Dalton, the woman was not responsible for her actions. There is no question that some women suffer from symptoms like Julia's that may be related to the repression of valuable input from the unconscious. And as we will discuss in more depth in Chapter Six, as women enter their thirties they tend to have more anovulatory cycles in which no egg is released, and therefore there is no corpus luteum to manufacture progesterone. Progesterone is required, in part, to offset some of the physiological effects of estrogen, and when it is lacking, symptoms like bloating, irritability, and confusion may result. Dr. Dalton has, in fact, treated some cases of PMS very successfully with natural progesterone suppositories. Yet, if we subscribe to the viewpoint that the normal "negativity" that surfaces premenstrually can escalate to craziness or violence, I believe we do a disservice to the physiological gift it represents in terms of alerting us to areas of our life that need attention so that we can remain in balance and in relationship harmony.

One study found that fewer than 20 percent of the women who volunteered to be studied met the criteria for PMS—moderate to severe physical or psychological symptoms for at least the six preceding menstrual cycles. Reviews of the literature consistently fail to find that PMS is a serious problem for most women, yet the myth persists that women as a whole are incapacitated by this syndrome. One of the most impressive things about the human body, however, is that discomfort is rarely wasted. It is usually part of a feedback system whose final goal is to restore homeostasis. If we adopt the increasingly well-documented point of view that the body runs on a system of subtle *chi* energy, in tune with a larger, universal energy source, the symptoms of PMS can be understood as a blockage of *chi*. Its occurrence can then be appreciated as part of a biological feedback loop that is meant to attract our attention to the question, "What is happening in my life—in the web of relationships to self, others, and the natural world, that is blocking the flow of energy and producing these symptoms?"

Psychophysiologist Margaret Altemus and her colleagues carried out a very interesting study of auditory perception and the menstrual cycle that bears on this question. They used a technique called the dichotic listening test, a neuropsychological measure of brain function. Different words were presented through headphones to the right and left ears of women both in the follicular phase of the cycle (before ovulation) and in the luteal phase (premenstrually). Sensory input to the brain is contralateral, so that a sound presented to the right ear feeds into the left hemisphere, which also happens to be the location of language processing. Words presented to the left ear are shunted to the right brain and then back to the left hemisphere where they are perceived as meaningful symbols.

In one part of the experiment emotionally charged words—either positive or negative—were paired with neutral words, one presented to each ear. Women in general showed a strong trend toward hearing fewer positive words premenstrually. But those who reported dysphoria (negative moods) premenstrually heard significantly fewer positive words compared to their performance in the follicular, or preovulatory, phase of the cycle. The authors interpret the results as indicating greater activation of the right hemisphere and a decline in left-brain function premenstrually. They state, "These results suggest that other aspects of right hemisphere function also may be enhanced premenstrually. Menstrual cycle research has tended to measure only negative aspects of the premenstrual period. Other measures may detect enhancement of more valued right hemisphere functions premenstrually, particularly in the group of women who experience more dysphoria."

One way to interpret these findings is that women experience and express emotions cyclically. As a society we tend to frown on negativity and like to deny the dark side of our emotions. Our brain and hormones, however, conspire to create a certain interval during each month when we are neurophysiologically less available for joy and more tuned in to the release of difficult emotions that may have been building up all month. This emotional housecleaning is wrongly viewed as bitchiness or complaining, but when seen rightly and heeded, it may be a valuable stress reducer and guide to what we need to change or pay attention to so that our lives will run more smoothly. This is the benefit to feeling down. Additionally, since intuitive capacity, empathy, and interdependent perception are also right-brain functions, it follows that the premenstrual and menstrual phases of our cycle are indeed times of enhanced wisdom.

One of the most august figures in the field of psychosomatic medicine, Dr. Larry LeShan, is a walking encyclopedia of studies—and just as important, studies that were never published because the researchers couldn't understand the data. Dr. LeShan told me of a study done in the biology department of William and Mary College in the mid-1940s that found a very interesting correlate to premenstrual moodiness. When menstrual mood changes were measured throughout the year, there were two clusters of high negativity that turned out to occur on the equinoxes—those two days each year when the hours of dark and light are equal. Since our pineal glands, which sense darkness and light, are intimately related to the onset of puberty and the monthly fluctuation of hormones, the modern researcher would have been fascinated with the correlation between light/dark cycles, hormones, and mood. But since these physiological pathways were incompletely understood fifty years ago when the study was made, the researchers considered their data "weird" and promptly scuttled it.

What does all this mean? Women are creatures of the natural world who by virtue of our physiology are deeply entrained to the rhythms of darkness and light, sun and moon. Our brains and hormones work in synchrony to make us more available to the wisdom that arises from interdependent perception during our menstrual flow and perhaps during the equinoxes. Discomfort and dysphoria can be interpreted as a positive signal to reflect so that we can make ourselves available to information coming in through many sensory channels—the "sixth sense" included.

The gifts of middle childhood build on the circuits of empathy, interdependent perception, and intuition that have been developing since a girl's birth. The ability to see relationships with clarity, the uncanny tendency to recognize instances of relational injustice and cry foul, and the development of the morality of the heart are remarkable female capacities that mark middle childhood. Puberty as the entrance into a cyclic bio-psycho-spiritual feedback loop that functions to preserve clarity, restore emotional balance and relational harmony, and attune to greater wisdom is an additional gift.

Julia's emergence from childhood to womanhood is an interesting, but confusing, time. Emotions run high, and she wonders whether telling the truth of how she feels is always the right thing to do. When she finally told her boyfriend that she thought he was cheating on her, he became irate, and they broke up. A few weeks later she found out that she was right after all, but she misses him nonetheless. Truth often upsets people and she has begun to notice that her mother, like many women, often avoids telling the truth to keep the peace. Can this be right? What of the toll it takes on relationships? Balancing the logic of the mind and the wisdom of the heart with the intuition that keeps her tuned in to the relational world is a gift that for Julia, like other adolescent girls in our culture, is a daunting challenge because she has so few role models to turn to.

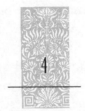

AGES 14–21: ADOLESCENCE

SNOW WHITE FALLS ASLEEP, BUT AWAKENS TO HERSELF

Fifteen-year-old Julia is sitting at the dinner table, glumly making designs with a pile of peas that she has been pushing around her plate for several minutes. Most of the meal remains untouched. Her eleven-year-old brother, Alex, is prattling on about the next game that will challenge the impressive lead that his Little League team has amassed this spring, but their mother's eyes are fixed on Julia. When there's a break in the conversation, she turns to her daughter and says, "Honey, I'm worried about you. You look tired and you're losing weight."

"Well, at least that's good." Julia snorts. "I'm too fat, Mom. My thunder thighs are the laugh of gym class. Summer's almost here, too, and I can't even think about wearing a bathing suit. And my face is breaking out." She points to a few pink spots on her chin. "Ugh, I *hate* myself," she finishes with a groan and lapses into silence.

Julia is an athlete who is five feet five inches tall and weighs one hundred and twenty-five pounds, firmly toned. She looks great. Her father, John, hastens to tell her so, adding that she's too hard on herself. Julia looks up from her peas with an angry glare. "What would you know? You don't go to my school. The popular girls all look like Kate Moss. I have to lose at least twenty pounds," she whines, exasperated.

"Yeah," observes Alex with an attempt at humor, "you do have kind of a chubby butt." This is the last straw. With tears gathering in the corners of her eyes, Julia growls, "May I *please* be excused," as she gets up out of her chair and stomps off to her room. A few minutes later she returns outfitted with jogging sneakers, a Walkman plugged in to her ears, glossy brown hair tied back in a ponytail, and a set of fluorescent ankle safety bands since it will be dark when she returns from her nightly five-mile run.

"Be careful," John calls. "Oh, Daddy." Julia places her hands on her hips and arranges her face into a perfect mask of disgust. "I'm not a baby. I can take care of myself." Then relenting a little she walks over to her parents, gives them both a peck on the cheek, and adds softly, "Stop worrying about me so much, you guys. Everybody has to grow up."

SNOW WHITE FALLS ASLEEP

In her best-selling book *Reviving Ophelia*, psychologist Mary Pipher writes, "Something dramatic happens to girls in early adolescence. Just as planes and ships disappear mysteriously into the Bermuda Triangle, so do the selves of girls go down in droves. They crash and burn in the developmental Bermuda Triangle. . . . Fairy tales capture the essence of this phenomenon. Young women eat poisoned apples or prick their fingers with poisoned needles and fall asleep for a hundred years."

Pipher's book title derives from the story of Shakespeare's Ophelia, who is happy and competent as a girl, but with the onset of adolescence, lives only for Hamlet's approval, thus losing herself. She serves as a symbol for the process through which charming, imaginative, perceptive, energetic young girls like Julia often become brooding, silent teenagers. This is not a new phenomenon. Shakespeare described it as did numerous psychologists who have generated a literature that stretches back to 1905, documenting the decrease in self-worth, plummeting assessment of body image, eating disorders, depression, and thoughts of suicide that characterize this age. Girls who were accomplished, exuberant, and outgoing in middle childhood often become unsure of themselves, depressed, and confused as adolescents. A variety of psychological and sociological theories have been invoked to explain this loss of self. In this chapter we will build on some of these theories, relating them to the maturation of the bio-psycho-spiritual feedback loop, and ultimately examining why falling asleep to self may be a natural part of a woman's cycle of awakening.

THE POWER TO BE OR THE POWER TO PLEASE

The adolescent drama of Snow White has been cast, through time, as a power issue, or rather as one of the relative powerlessness of women. Writers as diverse as Simone de Beauvoir and neo-Freudian Karen Horney believe that the adolescent girl's doubt and depression occur in tandem with her growing realization that women in our culture have little power other than to become adored, submissive appendages of men. When power is borrowed from learning to please a man, as Ophelia tries to please Hamlet, or as Julia tries to please would-be suitors by obsessing about her weight, the girl starts to lose track of some of her own talents and interests.

Central to this drama is an irreconcilable tension, a classic double bind where you are damned if you do and damned if you don't. To be successful as a person in her own right, a woman is expected to think and act like a man, yet she will always be thought of as inferior in a game run by male rules. Furthermore, the behavior of a successful woman is likely to be perceived as masculine and threatening, making it harder to enter into an intimate love relationship. The adolescent, who is expert at understanding the nuances of personal exchange, awakens from the charmed, outspoken period of middle childhood with a sudden, sickening awareness of this grown-up bind.

My mother, an educated woman who graduated from Boston University in the late 1920s, verbalized this bind in my own adolescent years with an unwelcome piece of advice. "You may be smart, Joani, but don't let the boys know it. Men are scared of smart women and you'll end up alone in your ivory tower." Her advice reminds me of the story of Rapunzel, locked in a tower by a witch, having to let her hair down as a rope in order to tryst with her lover. And what of Snow White? Her beauty and goodness were a challenge to the wicked queen, like Rapunzel's witch, a metaphor for the negative, aggressive, shadow side of masculinity that women fear within themselves. Fooled into eating a poisoned apple, Snow White fell into a deathlike sleep. She awakened only when a charming prince, allured by her beauty as she lay entombed in a glass coffin, kissed her and brought her back to life. The sinister message of this story, like that of Rapunzel, is that a woman's masculine aspect embodies death-dealing qualities. The apple of her wisdom is poisoned and her only hope of a good life is to attract a prince who admires her for the life-giving qualities of subservience, kindness, and feminine beauty. The roots of the young woman's desire to please a man, however, are biological as well as sociological, which may explain why this adolescent power bind can be a life-or-death drama for some young women.

THE SOCIOBIOLOGY OF BODY IMAGE

Julia, like many teenagers, has a consuming, self-centered focus on being attractive. Although some of her concern has certainly been engendered by advertisements, movies, television and the like, concerns about beauty are instinctual because they have to do with the strongest biological urge of all—sex and the continuation of the species. The rituals of courtship and mating may vary in different times and cultures, yet they follow a basic pattern that anthropologist Helen Fisher summarizes so well in her fascinating book, *Anatomy of Love*. Energetic, wide-hipped, plump, clear-skinned women are preferred by men of all cultures because these characteristics bode well for child-bearing potential. This preference is hardwired into the instinctual reptilian brain, whose main focus is survival. But as Julia knows, and tries to emulate, the current white female ideal of an attractive woman is the cadaverous model and hard-bodied movie star. Thin is in. And when social pressures buck biology, trouble brews.

A 1995 study at the University of Arizona found that 90 percent of white teenage girls were unhappy with their weight. These girls cited the statistics of a supermodel (5'7" and one hundred to one hundred ten pounds) as the ideal height and weight. Since the average American woman weighs one hundred forty-three pounds, and fewer than one quarter of American women are taller than 5'4", as my children often say, "Something is wrong with this picture." In 1994, 62 percent of white girls reported dieting. If medieval torture racks were for sale I have no doubt that many teenagers would flock to buy them in the hopes of becoming taller.

The irony of the battle of the bulge is that Julia's angst over thin thighs is actually wasted on the majority of males that she is trying so hard to attract. Boys polled at a midwestern high school found the spindly supermodel look "sickly" and "gross." Plump, healthy women are apparently a biological ideal that hasn't gone out of style because that template for attractiveness is programmed into ancient neuronal pathways designed for survival and procreation of the species. But white women, on the whole, can't shake the feeling that you can't be either too rich or too thin. Six months into a new relationship at the age of forty-nine (I'm 5'4" and generally weigh between one hundred fifteen and one hundred twenty pounds) I reminisced wistfully about my college weight of one hundred to one hundred five pounds. My husband-to-be was shocked. "Yuck, you must have looked awful. Don't you know that men don't like women with skinny legs?" He laughed, singing a song of that title. I wondered why I always thought they did and whether I'd ever be able to shake that cultural conditioning.

In contrast to white girls, the University of Arizona study not only found that 70 percent of black teenagers were satisfied with their bodies, but that 64 percent believed that it was better to be a little overweight than underweight. Furthermore, 65 percent said that women become more beautiful with age, whereas white girls believe that beauty fades. Even black girls who were significantly overweight rated themselves as happy. Most encouraging about black culture was the girls' sense that *beauty is an attitude* rather than an exterior characteristic. One of the study's coauthors, anthropologist Mimi Nichter, observed that the window of beauty is very small in white culture. It gets smaller, apparently, as we get older. A study by the American Association of University Women found that 60 percent of elementary school girls were happy with themselves. By high school only 30 percent were happy. The rest, like Julia, were lost somewhere in the thicket of harsh self-judgment.

Nearly 10 percent of American women, a statistic that swells to 20 percent during adolescence, starve themselves or binge and purge. Ninety to ninety-five percent of anorexics and bulimics are women. And anorexia is a potentially fatal illness. Five to fifteen percent of hospitalized anorexics die in treatment and only about 50 percent eventually recover. Although accounts of anorexia can be found as far back as 1825, researchers like Naomi Wolf believe that self-starvation picked up momentum in the 1920s when the angular outline of the flappers replaced the more curvaceous outlines of their predecessors. For the first time, women were entering the workforce in large numbers, and they adopted the physical characteristics of men. The urge for boyish-looking bodies has gathered momentum ever since. Models in my mother's generation weighed only 8 percent less than average; today's models weigh nearly 25 percent less. In 1951 Miss Sweden was 5'7" tall and weighed one hundred fifty-one pounds. In 1983 Miss Sweden was 5'9" tall and weighed one hundred nine pounds. And although models have grown thinner, the average American woman has gotten heavier since the fifties, creating an enormous discrepancy between the real and the ideal. Teenagers like Julia fall into the resultant body gap, losing self-esteem and confidence while yearning for bodies that were never meant to be.

THE NEUROBIOLOGY OF BODY IMAGE

The neurobiology of eating behavior provides a fascinating context for sociological concerns about body image. When neurosurgeon Wilder Penfield stimulated areas of patients' brains prior to surgery, he developed a detailed map of how the body is represented on the surface of the cortex. There are two such maps; one for touch (somatosensory) and the other for body movement (motor). These maps looks like distorted human bodies with some parts much larger or smaller than on an actual body, and are called *homunculi*, or "little people." The largest area of representation on both the sensory and motor homunculi is the jaw because we are mammals and the ability to suckle as infants is the single most important voluntary activity related to survival.

As babies, most of us are rewarded for eating. So, in addition to strengthening basic circuits in the sensory and motor areas of the cortex, eating behavior also creates sturdy myelinated pathways between the limbic system and the frontal lobes, carrying the message that eating is a socially acceptable activity that will bring us both pleasure and reward from loved ones. Julia, like many children, was raised as a charter member of the clean-plate club. Do you remember all those starving children in China or India who were used as incentives for you to finish your meal? They live on in your neural circuitry, compelling you to please your parents by eating, an activity that is intrinsically pleasurable in its own right. Not only does eating stimulate neurons in the medial forebrain bundle of the hypothalamus, the "pleasure center" of the brain, but it also sends messages from the limbic system to the frontal lobes along the tracts that Mommy and Daddy have thickened by praising us for eating when we were young. What could be more delightful than engaging in a biologically pleasurable activity that also triggers the feelings of security, self-confidence, self-esteem, and belonging that parental praise creates? If you think about a baby, blissfully suckling, rocked in loving arms, you'll get some sense of the powerful positive reinforcer that eating can be.

While we are rewarded for eating in early childhood, by adolescence many white girls like Julia have internalized the strong, conflicting message that eating is bad—it leads to fat. Social/biological binds are inherently stressful, particularly when they involve survival circuits like feeding. While doing a senior honors thesis at Bryn Mawr College in the 1960s, I conducted research at Wyeth Laboratories in the pharmaceutical research division. The project involved control of feeding behavior and centered on a particular group of neurons in the hypothalamus called the ventromedial nucleus (VMN). If this area is destroyed an animal loses control of appetite and becomes obese. It turns out that the VMN is also the site of female sexual arousal. Thus, sex and feeding are intimately related. The fact that many girls who are sexually abused in childhood and adolescence subsequently become obese may be more complex than the frequently cited hypothesis that excess weight is a kind of armor, an unconscious attempt to avoid further exploitation. The close proximity of neurons that control weight to those that mediate sexual arousal may provide a biological basis for the weight gain. Sexual issues have also been linked to self-starvation. One theory of anorexia suggests that pubescent girls who are afraid to grow up and become sexual starve themselves to delay puberty or stop their periods.

THE POLITICS OF SELF-STARVATION

The problem with all current explanations of anorexia, including those based on biology, societal values, or familial dysfunction, is that they are insufficient to explain the preponderance of anorexia in upper-middle-class white girls. Self-starvation tends to be almost exclusively an affliction of particularly bright, privileged young women. Psychologist Catherine Steiner-Adair suggests an interesting anthropologically based model that accommodates these sociological findings. She writes, "Universally, the rounded female body has symbolically represented the value of relationships in life, the interrelatedness and interdependency of people. The most obvious symbol is that of the full-breasted, wide-hipped, and pregnant 'Great Mother.'" She likens anorexia to an unconscious hunger strike in which the adolescent female is making a political protest against a society that has turned its back on the primacy of relationship and interrelatedness, devaluing core feminine values that are central to the adolescent girl's identity. The starved, emaciated female becomes a stark symbol of a starved, degenerate culture that provides the young woman few role models to internalize in the process of forging a strong identity based on self-in-relation to others.

FINDING AN IDENTITY

Julia has butterflies in her stomach as she steps out of her friend Amber's car and wonders whether her parents are at home. Her hand moves fleetingly toward her nose, which still stings from the little gold ring that has just been inserted at a jeweler's in the mall. Torn between allegiance to her friends, two of whom have just undergone the same initiation, and to her parents, who she feels sure will "throw a nutty," Julia is suspended in a maelstrom of conflicting feelings. She feels both proud of her independence and guilty for betraying her family's conservative values. She feels like a woman, and simultaneously like a bad little girl. Gathering courage to walk into the house, Julia instinctively settles on anger as the emotion most useful for surviving the expected onslaught. The problem is that unlike her brother, Alex, Julia has trouble expressing anger, and is more likely to become penitent and submissive during confrontations in an attempt to restore the peace. "If they gave Alex heat about an earring," she thinks, "he'd insist on being his own person and then stomp off, slam his bedroom door, and play his stereo at about a zillion decibels. I wish I could do that, but I'm such a wimp. I'll probably just knuckle under and pull the stupid thing out."

Alex turns out to be the only one in the kitchen when Julia strides in with a false sense of bravado. Absorbed in a tuna fish sandwich, he is oblivious to his sister's nose. Disappointed with the lack of notice, Julia calls his attention to her new symbol of independent identity. His face breaks into a big grin, "Hey, that's really sick," he opines, by way of compliment. "Mom and Dad will ground you for sure." Julia has considered this possibility carefully since her best friend, Gwen, is still grounded two weeks after a lip piercing whose only evidence is a small red mark where the little hole has closed since her mother made her throw away the gold ring. Gwen is furious at her mother for grounding her, and madder still at her father, who never voices his own opinion now that he and her mother are divorced. Like many adolescent girls, Gwen expresses her anger indirectly through various acts of quiet rebellion. She has been sexually active since fifteen, like 15 percent of her female peers, and uses sexual promiscuity as a covert way to express anger at her parents, while getting at least a temporary sense of peace and belonging from her boyfriends. Unlike Gwen, if Julia is grounded she won't act out sexually; she is more likely to become withdrawn and spend her time in solitary pursuits like running and reading. Both girls have trouble expressing opinions and negative feelings, and they have chosen different outlets.

When Sylvia and John come home from visiting friends, they are surprised and less than delighted about their daughter's nose ring, but they know better than to alienate her. Julia is a responsible child, and their main concern is that she is easily discouraged and gives up when the things she wants are not easy to come by. The discussion centers on their sad feelings that she didn't trust them enough to discuss the idea before taking the plunge, and a respectful inquiry about why Julia wanted the piercing. Their honesty, and the fact that they are discussing how her behavior made them feel, rather than blaming her, opens the way for Julia to talk about her own angry and hurt feelings. She has been rejected by a clique of girls to whom she had been close since grammar school, because of a growing values gap. She likes basketball and track and they prefer to party. Julia has resolved her misery by finding a new peer group whose values include classical music, physical fitness, and nose rings as an odd touch seemingly inspired by a desire not to appear stodgy. Because of her parents' trust, and their dedication to respectful communication, Julia gets to keep her nose ring. She also gets some practice in expressing her feelings, especially anger.

LOSING OUR VOICES

If Julia does not find her own voice, she will be at risk for continuing in the role of peacekeeper, habitually giving up her own opinions and desires to keep relationships running smoothly. Her decision not to party with her old friends, even though it would have kept the peace and retained the old web of relationships, was an important step in developing an authentic sense of self. Getting the nose ring was a symbol of solidarity with a new group, and a reminder of her inner strength. Gwen, on the other hand, has been silenced both by a culture that hypes beauty and sexuality as a ticket to belonging, and by parents who did not bother to listen to the story behind the lip ring before summarily grounding their daughter. For Gwen, the act of body piercing told a story of feeling lost; for Julia it told a story of feeling found.

Psychologist Lyn Mikel Brown, who is part of a Harvard research team with Carol Gilligan, writes about how powerful it would be for an adolescent to have the opportunity to tell her own personal story in a ritualized way, just as she was standing on the brink of initiation into womanhood. When I was a junior in high school I tried to do something similar. I sat down one day and wrote out the story of my life in which I expressed deep dismay that my mother and I were on different wavelengths. She wanted me to grow up and marry a doctor, to be a rich and powerful man's wife. I didn't want to borrow a man's power, but to find my own—to be the doctor rather than marry him. The only way to make my mother happy was to focus on my appearance, which in her eyes always fell short of the mark. I never measured up to her standards, nor did she appreciate that mine might be different.

I came home from school one day to the sound of fury. My mother had found my story, invaded my privacy by reading it, and was deeply wounded. Hadn't she done her best for me, given me everything? She couldn't understand how a girl with so much felt so empty, so she told me that I was not entitled to feel as I did. I was a spoiled, ungrateful child who should be ashamed of myself. We did not speak, other than to communicate about necessities, for a month. We did not speak about feelings for another thirty years. The unfortunate consequence of having my story ridiculed rather than acknowledged, was that I formed a dangerous identity. Rather than becoming Joani, I defined myself as being not-Lillian—not like my mother. She was aggressive so I became a people pleaser. She went to the beauty parlor weekly so I grew my hair down to my waist. She was obsessed with clothes, so I dressed like a hippie.

Whereas I lost parts of myself through a negative identification, many adolescents lose themselves in a positive identification with a cultural norm that casts women as submissive peacemakers. We are socialized progressively to be nice, to please others, and not to ask embarrassing questions or raise difficult issues. This conditioning creeps up during adolescence, silencing the girl who was vocal in middle childhood, the girl whose ease with the relational world led her to tell the truth about what she saw and heard in the arena of human relationships. At ten Julia would watch her mother's body language and ask why she was angry. If Sylvia denied her feelings, her daughter would doggedly insist on the truth. She knew what she knew and had no hesitation about voicing her perceptions and prying until she got an honest answer. But at sixteen, Julia has learned a new set of rules. People wear masks that hide their feelings. Women retreat behind meaningless statements like "How interesting" and "I'm fine, how are you?" And it's not polite to pull down a mask, so just look the other way.

One of the unspoken rules of adult feminine behavior is that we must buffer strife, even at the expense of submerging our own feelings. When the adolescent learns this rule, she runs the risk of becoming a "psychic sponge" for the negative emotions of family and friends. Furthermore, she may have few outlets through which to discharge the accumulated stress. Alcoholic parents, for example, may go merrily on their way while their adolescent daughter, bent on keeping the peace, grapples with their problems symbolically in her dreams or develops an ulcer. I believe that young women—who have opened to a deep dimension of intuition at puberty—are flooded with psychic impressions of other people's pain that they then act out as their own. The central developmental question of a girl's adolescence becomes "Where do I begin and other people end?" Other ways of posing this question might be "Where are my boundaries?" or "Can I take care of my own needs and still maintain relationships with others?" One of the best statements of this bind, and a delightful allegory of its resolution, are contained in the classic story of Heidi, which is about a little girl who was finally able to find her own identity, her own voice.

HEIDI: A GIRL FINDS HER VOICE

Heidi is a story that warms the heart because it focuses on the archetype of redemption. Heidi's grandfather, a bitter, angry, isolated old man is reborn through the innocent love of a small child, and a crippled girl by the name of Clara learns to walk. But it is Heidi's own redemption—her courageous act of becoming more fully a person—that gives this story special importance to women. If you haven't seen the classic movie adaptation starring Jason Robards and Jessica Lange recently, you might enjoy it as a tale that highlights the unique feminine gifts of relationality and nurture, and the adolescent (and sometimes lifetime) struggle to balance giving to others with caring for ourselves.

Heidi was a precocious, resilient child who exuded love in spite of being orphaned at an early age, brought to a remote village in the Swiss Alps to live with a bitter grandfather who initially rejected her, and finally forming a loving relationship with her grandfather and an ex-tended family only to be sold into servitude as a companion for the rich, crippled, lonely Clara who lived in Frankfurt. After a year of liv-ing with Clara, who came to love and depend on the bright, cheerful, and compassionate little girl as the center of her life, Heidi became dangerously depressed. Her own life had been sacrificed to the needs of another, and she was pining away for her family in the Alps, having repetitive dreams that her best friend, Peter's, grandmother, a woman she also called Grandmother, was dying. Out of concern for Heidi's failing health, Clara's family finally allowed her to return to her beloved Alps for a month-long visit.

When Heidi arrived home, Grandmother was indeed dying. In a touching deathbed scene, the old woman told Heidi that her capacity to love and bring such joy into the lives of others was both a gift and a curse. Grandmother had, in fact, articulated the developmental dilemma of adolescence—how a young girl, skilled in empathetic rela-tionality, must learn to care for herself without feeling selfish when she cannot meet the needs of others. She extracted a promise from Heidi, one that the little girl was not yet able to comprehend, a solemn vow to claim her own happiness rather than living as a wish-fulfiller for oth-ers.

At the end of the month, Clara and her family came to visit for a few days before bringing Heidi back to Frankfurt. She and Peter managed to carry the crippled Clara to a high mountain pasture where the housebound invalid could experience the remarkable charms of the Alps firsthand. There in the pristine beauty—at the center of her spir-itual/emotional universe—Heidi had a revelation. Clara began to dis-cuss their return to Frankfurt and Heidi realized that her happiness was there in the Alps, not in continuing to be an object of comfort for Clara in Frankfurt. As she haltingly spoke this difficult truth, the crippled Clara went into a self-centered frenzy that culminated in Heidi's losing her footing and falling over a cliff. Dangling precariously from a sapling that had broken her fall, Heidi was ultimately rescued by Peter and Clara, who had to will her crippled legs to move in order to participate in saving her friend's life.

Heidi's courageous decision to disappoint Clara by choosing to stay in the mountains and claim her own happiness was the fulfillment of her promise to Grandmother. Her falling over the cliff and needing to be rescued also demonstrates an important principle vital to a woman's development of authentic compassion. When we compulsively take care of other people it leaves them disempowered, unaware of their own strengths. But when we insist that they stand up on their own and take care of themselves, they have an opportunity to find their power. In this way both they and we are redeemed.

SELF VERSUS OTHERS

Writing of her detailed observations of adolescent girls negotiating relationship, Carol Gilligan observes that "To seek connection with others by excluding oneself is a strategy destined to fail. . . . Yet teenage girls and adult women often seem to get caught on the horns of a dilemma: is it better to respond to others and abandon themselves or to respond to themselves and abandon others? The dilemma is one of 'being a good woman, or . . . being selfish.'"

According to Erik Erikson, the developmental crisis of late adolescence for both girls and boys is *intimacy versus isolation*. But, as we've discussed, the establishment of intimate relationships has been a major focus of girls' development since infancy. Boys who have been busy learning autonomy and separation up to this point must now learn the lessons of gaining affection and interdependence on which true intimacy is based, while girls must grapple with the developmental crisis that Gilligan described. We must become bridgers and balancers, learning to care for ourselves as much as we care for others.

This task of balancing depends on the development of a skill that psychologist Janet Surrey calls "relationship-authenticity," a style of communication that is purposeful, emotionally real, connected, clear, and vital. Intimate relationship requires the ability to risk sharing one's full range of emotions and challenging old patterns of dishonesty or the avoidance of feelings. Distinctly different from attachment, intimacy requires an honest give and take—a willingness to be present to the stories in one's own body and to share that information with the other.

Julia, at twenty, is a sophomore at the University of Vermont. Distressed by the subtle flirtatiousness of her professor while discussing a term paper in political science, she is forthright in her response. "I feel very uncomfortable when you stand so close to me, would you please move back and give me a little more space." He does, and although she has risked disapproval by clearly stating her boundaries, the incident passes and they resume their previous relationship roles. A Julia whose parents had been less emotionally understanding and honest with their feelings as she was growing up might have responded differently. If her boundaries were too permeable she could have ended up in an unwanted sexual liaison. If her boundaries were too rigid she might have overreacted and created an unnecessary scene. A girl's relationship to her mother is critically important in this regard. If we feel seen by our mothers, and free to engage in the give-and-take of honest exchange, a pattern of relationship authenticity is set. In my own case, the lack of honest communication with my mother was a stumbling block to setting healthy boundaries that took years to overcome, with the result that intimate relationships with men were difficult. Either I felt taken advantage of because I couldn't state my own needs, or I felt so threatened that I would wall myself off and end the relationship.

Real intimacy with a person of the opposite sex, says Erikson, requires a firmly developed sense of gender and personal identity. This requires both the ability to fuse with another, to let down boundaries in some areas of our life while holding on to them in others. For example, Julia may be ready to let down emotional barriers and share her goals, dreams, wounds, and hopes with her boyfriend, but she may not wish to let down sexual boundaries. If a young woman's boundaries are healthy, like Julia's, she can differ from another person in likes, behaviors, and habits without undue conflict. She doesn't need to conform to the other in order to feel safe from rejection and there is no need to force the other to conform to her. This mutual respect of self and other is the cornerstone of intimacy, the prerequisite for mature love.

THE HEART OF A WOMAN, THE BRAIN
OF A CODEPENDENT

The emotional development that occurs during adolescence parallels the myelination of specific pathways in the brain that are important for logical, abstract, symbolic thought. Jean Piaget theorized that adolescence was characterized by the capacity for formal/abstract thinking. By this time we can think our own thoughts—we have opinions that are separable from other people's, we can group concepts and calculate probabilities, and we can stand back and reflect on ourselves. If you've ever seen the early Woody Allen films, when a voice inside his head offers constant comments on his behavior, you can relate to what Piaget means by self-reflection.

Self-reflective capacities are probably related to the myelination of association areas in the adolescent brain that are important for calculating probabilities and thinking symbolically. The frontal lobes, the so-called "heart of the brain," are continuing to mature at the same time, laying down templates for social comportment—in other words, the ability to inhibit behaviors that would be socially inappropriate. For example, some people suffer from an unfortunate kind of seizure in the frontal lobe called Tourette's syndrome. When a seizure occurs they have facial tics and involuntarily swear a blue streak. Social sanctions have been temporarily short-circuited and inappropriate actions are released from inhibition.

During the time that the frontal lobes are busily embroidering what is socially acceptable into myelinated pathways, the adolescent female is straddling the horns of the nice-versus-selfish dilemma. If she decides that the most acceptable behavior is to scuttle her own needs in favor of other people's, her decision is likely to become a permanent frontal lobe reality. The resultant biopsychological feedback loop supports a serious personality disorder called codependency, a loss of self in which other people's needs are considered primary. The codependent will overwork herself, worry continually over the needs and behaviors of others, and deny her own needs—a pattern that can lead to anger, resentment, burnout, depression, addiction, and stress-related illness.

The frustration of losing oneself is stored in the body as a story of victimization—of reaching out in relationship only to be wounded and rejected. The old twelve-step definition of a codependent is funny, but cuts right to the bone—a codependent is a person who, at the moment of her death, sees someone else's life flash in front of her eyes. A codependent Julia having sex for the first time might be more interested in whether her suitor was pleased than whether her own needs were met. She would be unlikely to observe "I know it was good for him, but was it good for me?" If it wasn't good for her she certainly wouldn't bring it up. Instead, she'd be likely to fake orgasm and begin a pattern of sexual self-denial that would progressively deaden her ability to experience pleasure.

SNOW WHITE WAKES UP:
THE GIFT OF ADOLESCENCE

If we manage to exit adolescence with the proper balance of caring for self and others, we extend the empathy that we developed in early and middle childhood to ourselves. The resultant skills of authenticity then bring greater awareness to both partners in a relationship, elevating it to a spiritual level where each person can grow in sensitivity, confidence, creativity and self-esteem. Janet Surrey calls these psychospiritual skills of relationship authenticity the "core self" of a woman.

The development of a core self, a strong yet pliable identity in which the previous gifts of relationality, intuition, and the logic of the heart are combined in a conscious way bestows life's most precious spiritual gift—the ability to relate to both self and others with true intimacy. Unfortunately, it is the rare adolescent today who grows up in a home like Julia's where her parents recognize that the silent, brooding years during which their charming daughter falls asleep like Snow White are a time of metamorphosis during which their child is in a kind of cocoon from which she will emerge transformed if models of authentic relationship are available to her.

The time of menarche, when our periods first come, and our bodies take on the shape of a woman, are an obvious metamorphosis. But they are accompanied by a no less stunning psychological and spiritual metamorphosis during the subsequent seven-year cycle. Gilligan's group has found that young girls tend to lose their voices just before the time of puberty, in the fourth and fifth grades, when they openly state that they have learned that telling the truth is silly, dangerous, or in other ways uncomfortable. They have effectively entered a cocoon in which they are separated from the simple, nourishing relationality of middle childhood. Julia at sixteen, for example, is a changeling whose world has undergone a dramatic shift in a few short years. During middle childhood her family, and the inner fantasy world she expressed through her dolls, crayons, and games of make-believe were the center of existence and the source of her identity. But suddenly she is confronted with a troubling, unfair, and confusing world that is unpredictable, and where love does not always win out. Even your friends can turn on you, depriving you of a precious link to the world outside, a lifeline to hold on to while crossing the sea of change. Since having friends is critical to staying afloat, identification with a peer group ranks right up there with survival issues like food and shelter.

For many adolescent girls in the inner city, having a baby establishes the teenager as a woman on her own, part of a tribe of other single women with children. In some suburbs, experimentation with alcohol and drugs or getting tattoos forges looser but similar bonds. The teenagers have devised rites of passage—initiation rituals—that are symbols of their solidarity and the safety they provide for one another during the time of metamorphosis. A nose ring was a sign of belonging for Julia, a lifeline similar to the tattered blanket that she once dragged to kindergarten as a way of feeling at home in a new place. For her parents the nose ring was not evidence that Julia had gone over the edge and had to be punished or restrained. It was an invitation to relationship authenticity in which they passed the fruits of their own bio-psycho-spiritual development on to their daughter.

Julia had the good fortune to awaken from her sleep by the end of adolescence and exit from the cocoon having regained her voice and recognized that when one is self-full, true to her own perceptions, opinions, and needs, she doesn't have to fear being selfish. When we are self-full, we are also soulful. Our inherent relationality, intuition, and compassion guide us to act within the spiritual boundaries of self-in-relation. In that frame of reference the idea of self versus others is not a matter of who wins versus who loses. As in the story of Heidi, everyone wins as their own uniqueness is given the room to flower.

My belief is that there are relatively few Heidis or Julias in our culture. There is no map to lead us on the search for self-fulness as there used to be in cultures and societies that handed down a legacy of stories to their young. There are few role models of self-full, soulful women for our daughters to emulate, and in truth, many women are in midlife before they reclaim their voices. Some of us remain silenced throughout the life cycle, stuck in a state of arrested development. How might things have been different if the deeper meaning of Heidi's journey had been explained to us and then followed with some ritual, or rite of initiation, as potent as Heidi's vow to her dying grandmother? How might we make things different for our daughters, granddaughters, nieces, students, and young friends? It is time to reinvent our understanding of adolescence so that young women can combine their voices at an earlier time to bring the remarkable gifts of the feminine into a world that has never needed them more.

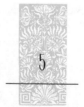

AGES 21–28: A HOME OF ONE'S OWN

THE PSYCHOBIOLOGY OF MATING
AND MOTHERHOOD

Julia is now a Peace Corps volunteer of twenty-three, halfway through a two-year assignment in Bangladesh where she is helping to run a birth control and childbirth education program for some of the poorest women in the world. She has taken to wearing colorful saris, and looks like a beautiful flower, as at the end of a long day she rests in a natural hammock, woven from the tangled aerial roots of an enormous, aged banyan tree. The sun is setting, and a shepherd is driving home his water buffalo, visible on the hill above her in dark silhouette against a fiery sky. As she breathes in the sweet scent of jasmine planted around the simple clinic, her body begins to relax. Just as she's about to float off on a daydream, a deep musical voice interrupts her reverie.

"Hello, I'm Roger Sanderson," he offers in a soft Georgia drawl, "are you Julia Macleish?" Julia stretches languidly and opens her eyes, greeted by a short, muscular man with a warm smile. She smiles in return, rising to a sitting position, and looks appraisingly at the ruggedly handsome young physician who has been assigned to the clinic for a three-month rotation. "Hi there, we weren't expecting you until tomorrow. It's great to have you here," she welcomes him, holding out her hand for his firm yet gentle clasp. In less than a minute, Julia has already formed an opinion of Roger. He's kind, attractive, and will be easy to work with. Her upturned nose, dusted with just the faintest trace of freckles, makes a charming little twitch as she gets up to show her new colleague around. They will, she senses, become good friends. And, she already hopes, perhaps something more.

THE BIOLOGY OF MATING: INFATUATION AND ATTRACTION

Roger and Julia are instantly attracted to each another, and over the next month that attraction increases to the point where nearly every waking hour is taken up with thoughts of each other. They work together, eat together, and take long walks in the countryside, sharing their life stories, their hopes, and dreams. They seem to exist in a cocoon, out of time, in which the rest of the world takes a backseat to their growing relationship. Whereas both of them had previously felt tired from workdays that could stretch to twelve or fourteen hours, they now seemed infused with superhuman energy, performing their clinical tasks efficiently and cheerfully. At the end of the day they are still energized, so the two stay up long into the night talking, and are soon lovers. Their lovemaking is long and gentle, often repeated two or three times in the course of an evening, nearly every night. And yet when morning comes, no matter how little sleep they've gotten, they are once again energized, wide-eyed, and ready to give their best. Too bad that infatuation can't be bottled!

Anthropologist Helen Fisher has written a fascinating account of infatuation, mating, marriage and divorce in her brilliant book, *Anatomy of Love.* When our mental map of a suitable mate coincides with periods of loneliness or readiness, and the pheromones in his sweat fit our biological fancy, we are primed for that peculiar altered state of lovesick obsession that we wish could last forever. But in several months the trance lifts and the moment of truth arrives. We are then left either to scratch our heads and wonder what could ever have seemed so cute about the way he strewed crumbs over the bed, or our body and mind downshift out of the unsustainable high of infatuation into the comfortable, stable, cuddly, and secure state called attachment.

Fisher traces the neurobiology of love beginning with a fascinating experiment centering on male armpit musk. The researchers collected pads they had asked male volunteers to wear under their arms. The sweat was then extracted with alcohol and the resultant odorless elixir dabbed under the noses of female volunteers. This male essence actually regularized the length of menstrual periods for those women whose cycles tended to be longer or shorter than average. Like amoebae flowing toward a food source, women may be unconsciously drawn to men because of the biological urge to maintain normal menstrual cycling. Women, too, produce pheromones that are capable of entraining other women into the same menstrual cycle—an oft-described phenomenon that Julia and her friends had noticed in their college dormitory.

In addition to the powerful effect of odorless pheromones, the particular scent of a man also plays a role in the mating game. Claus Wedekind, a zoologist at Bern University in Switzerland, discovered that women have strong preferences about whose armpits they sniff, unconsciously choosing men whose major histocompatibility (MHC) genes are different from their own. MHC genes leave their signature as proteins on the cell surface, and are critically important to the mechanisms through which the immune system recognizes our own cells and mounts attacks on invaders. Wedekind studied forty-nine women at the midpoint of their menstrual cycle (near the time of ovulation), when our sense of smell is keenest. Forty-four men were issued clean T-shirts and asked to wear them to bed for two nights. The shirts were then deposited in plastic-lined boxes with holes in the top. The women got to sniff seven samples: one clean T-shirt as a control, three from men with similar MHC genes and three from men with dissimilar genes. The latter group was judged most pleasant. Nature, as usual, is most clever in arranging our attractions to ensure the well-being of the species. Just how clever was revealed by geneticist Carole Ober of the University of Chicago. Ober studied Hutterites, a close-knit religious group who marry within their own community and do not practice contraception. She found that couples with similar MHC genes had fewer pregnancies and more miscarriages, suggesting that the immune system may be more likely to abort fetuses that carry similar MHC genes from both parents.

Outbreeding is generally advantageous for all organisms, a fact referred to as hybrid vigor. MHC differences may both increase fertility and produce offspring with hardier immune systems—a biological fact that only the nose knows. Women in Wedekind's study were often more than lukewarm about the T-shirts, rating some odors as beautiful and others as absolutely dreadful. But there was no one odor that suited all sniffers. Once again the reptilian brain, sometimes referred to as the rhinencephalon or smell brain, brings us back to the humble realization that our clever neocortical abilities to think and self-reflect are driven by pathways far more primitive and compelling than logic. The question women often ask, "Why am I so attracted to that guy—he's not at all my type?" may have a partial answer when we consider the hidden strength of the instinctual brain.

Women and men both respond to biological cues from potential partners. Wedekind chose to study men's musk for the simple reason that unshaved armpits are a better source of odor. It's a good bet that men respond to women's odors with similar attraction and repulsion. But odor is one of many cues that determine attraction. Taking a lesson from the birds and the bees, perhaps even certain tones of voice might resonate with our bodies. Julia, for example, was instantly taken by the musical quality of Roger's southern drawl. Female birds, after all, respond to the mating songs of males with increased heart rate and ovulation. But his song alone may not be enough to seal the union. Birds maintain territories and the more real estate the male controls, the likelier the female is to respond to his courtship songs. But even the right nest and the most beautiful warble isn't enough if the unfortunate male is funny looking. The female instinctually realizes that odd looks may be the harbingers of odd genes. To ensure the best for her offspring, she will only respond to good-looking warblers who have the potential to be good providers. Female birds also reward persistent courters, perhaps because they are demonstrating more stamina.

All in all, attraction and mating in the bird world is easier than in the human world because, on top of instincts, human beings are Homo sapiens, "wise beings." We think, and our limbic brain and neocortex can modify, and sometimes override, survival circuits. The woman who is attracted to a man whose voice and smell are right, but whose emotional maturity or other characteristics are not, can make a decision. After asking the question, "Why am I so attracted to this guy even though I'm picking up danger signals that he might be abusive, an addict, or a person that I'm going to have to take care of rather than having a mutually interdependent relationship with," a woman has two choices. She can leave, as Julia would be likely to do, or she can stay on and deny her own needs to become the caretaker of a wounded male. Like an egg that is biologically programmed to mend a damaged sperm, some women likewise feel compelled to heal wounded men. Codependency is apparently unheard of in the bird world. Only human females will choose mates they have to fix up, ignoring the instinctual urge that places good genes and survival of the fittest first in choosing a mate. Perhaps we should take a lesson from our bird sisters. Could it be that the proverbial suitor who keeps sending candy and flowers, the man who opens doors and holds your coat, the man who is patient through the dance of approach and avoidance that marks the beginning of some relationships, is better husband and father material? Perhaps he is biologically more inclined to hang in through the long winters and dark times that all long-term relationships go through.

But long before we know a man well enough for our neocortex to make the determination that he is emotionally healthy, suitable voice tone and smell send strong mating signals to the limbic system where a neurotransmitter called phenylethylamine, or PEA is released—and infatuation strikes. Within one minute of meeting Roger, Julia's rhinencephalon and limbic system were going into mating gear, setting the stage for the peculiar suspension of reason known as being love blind. In this state, she would have had trouble picking up cues about emotional unsuitability, because the more powerful instinctual circuits were still overriding reason.

PEA produces a wild, euphoric, amphetaminelike high that relieves depression and anxiety. You feel supercharged and filled with unaccustomed confidence. And rest, who needs rest? It's no trouble at all to leave work and drive for eight hours to meet your beloved in a motel in Yonkers in the dead of the night. Even if you normally have the sex drive of a doorpost, PEA shifts your libido into overdrive. Normally asleep by ten, you can make love all night long and then appear bright and cheerful for work in the morning like Roger and Julia. It is obvious that PEA is nature's way of ensuring the continuation of the species. You feel sexy, exhilarated, creative, optimistic, and charming. The world is your oyster. No obstacle seems too big to overcome.

PEA is also a temporary cure for shyness—the relational molecule par excellence. He's sooo easy to talk to, right? It's as if you've known one another for eons, lifetimes. He must be your soul mate. In no time at all you've exchanged your life stories and reached a deep under-standing. You feel that you can be fully yourself, loved for who you are. In the blissful glow of a limbic system soaked in PEA, his wounds and inadequacies just make him more adorable. Your wounds engender a fierce protectiveness in him. The moderating voices of your friends fall on deaf ears. "But he's unemployed and beat his last three wives." You respond, "That's because no one ever understood him before. He's so gentle and vulnerable. He just needs to be loved." In some way, PEA seems to decorticate normally perceptive, logical human beings.

If, after infatuation fades and the PEA supply diminishes, we find that our beloved is indeed a treasured partner, relationship proceeds to the cuddly, secure attachment phase, which has a neurobiology all of its own, mediated by endorphins. These naturally occurring pain re-lievers help anesthetize the couple to life's uncertainties and provide a modicum of biochemical security. While this usually occurs within three to six months, the process took longer for Julia and Roger, since he was transferred to southern India when his three-month rotation was over. Julia promptly fell back on transitional objects like pictures, letters, and a bouquet of dried bougainvillea that Roger had presented her with the day after they made love for the first time, to feel con-nected with her beloved. His absence, broken by occasional visits over the next year, sustained the state of infatuation. It was not until they returned to America, fourteen months after meeting, that their rela-tionship finally made the shift from infatuation to attachment. They rented an apartment together in Boston where Roger had been offered a position in the Department of Obstetrics and Gynecology at a Boston hospital, and where Julia began work on a degree in social work at a local college.

Relationship is not only physiological and psychological, it is also spiritual. During infatuation we are given a glimpse of what "holy" matrimony can be. The partners think the best of one another and through the resulting kindness and encouragement bring each other more fully into being. Shy people flower and confidence soars. Sex, too, is usually an experience of deep communion in the beginning. Even inexperienced partners can bring pleasure to one another when PEA has temporarily dropped the barriers around our hearts and two have become as one.

Infatuation is a kind of grace, a gift that we receive without having worked for it. But after the grace period is over, relationship requires work. For Julia and Roger, this work was a pleasure as they got to know one another better, made common friends and learned to make compromises that left time for relationship in their two busy schedules. To the delight of their parents, they married after having lived together for almost two years. A love relationship with a mate, however, is only part of a lifetime course in loving. Friends, co-workers, parents and other family, and even strangers, round out the curriculum.

MOTHERHOOD: TO BE OR NOT TO BE, CONTRACEPTION AND ABORTION

Betty Laverdure, an Ojibwa elder, shares traditional Native American wisdom about the choice to mother, "It was a privilege to have children, it was not a right. The elders, the women, they used to determine even who could have children. Had abortion medicines. And if somebody was abusing a child, they took that child, and the woman couldn't have children anymore. They determined that. Children are sacred. They are living treasures, gifts from the Great Spirit. You always treated them as if they didn't belong to you; they belonged to the Creator."

The sacred nature of motherhood has not always been as clearly communicated. When I was a little girl we used to skip rope to the rhyme, "First comes love, then comes marriage, then comes Joani (or Sally or Julia) with a baby carriage." This was the expected pattern, whether or not the woman was emotionally competent to bear children. While it might have been the dominant motif in the fifties when I was growing up, many women now have children without being married, and many married women (about 20 percent) don't have chil-

dren. And a surprisingly large number of women who become pregnant will never bear that child. Due to variety of circumstances, they
must make the difficult choice to abort.

Recent statistics indicate that 6.4 million American women become
pregnant each year. Only 44 percent of these pregnancies, or 2.8 million are intended; the majority are due to failures in contraception.
Nonetheless, about 4 million women give birth each year. Another 1.6
million have abortions. A statistic that shocked me was the fact that 47
percent of U.S. women will have had an abortion by the time they are
forty-five. In contrast to the pain of an unwanted pregnancy is that of a
woman who wants a child desperately but is unable to conceive or
carry a pregnancy to term. Seven and a half million women—about 13
percent of us of reproductive age—are infertile or have significant difficulties bearing children. Of those, about 2.3 million couples seek help
for infertility each year.

Rachel Benson Gold and Corey L. Richards compiled these statistics
in an effort to improve women's reproductive health. A colleague of
theirs at the Alan Guttmacher Institute, Jacqueline Darroch Forrest,
produced an excellent time line of a woman's reproductive life to help
determine health-care needs at different parts of our life cycle. She
computed the median age of typical events in a woman's reproductive
life and came up with the following sequence:

12.5 years: menarche
17.4 years: first intercourse
26.0 years: first birth
30.0 years: completion of family size
48.4 years: menopause

When I found myself pregnant at twenty-two, I became one of the
many women who, in technical terms, suffered a "failure" of contraception. My son Justin sneaked into the world past an ill-fitting di-
aphragm. (39.8 percent of married women between twenty and
twenty-four have the same experience with diaphragms, a rather
alarming statistic that I might have expected my gynecologist to
know.) At the time I was supporting our family on a meager graduate
student stipend while my husband alternately attended college and
volunteered as an "advance man" for Eugene McCarthy's unsuccessful

bid for the presidency. Politics and science made strange bedfellows, particularly coupled with my husband's long absences. After only a year together our marriage was already beginning to crumble. The added strain of laboratory research for my dissertation, in addition to the usual second-year medical curriculum, promised to keep me at school most evenings and weekends throughout the pregnancy. Nonetheless, I wanted to be a mother.

Although I sympathize deeply with women who choose abortion for a host of compelling reasons, it was not an option for me emotionally at that time. From the moment I realized that a child was growing in my womb, I felt a bond with that new life. My impending motherhood was announced to me over the phone, and it was indeed a shock. But after a minute or two of complete silence on my end, during which I was absorbing the information, I immediately switched into motherhood gear, wondering if I needed prenatal vitamins. I said to the doctor, supplements in mind, "My God, I'm pregnant. Is there anything I can do about it?" He immediately assumed that I wanted an abortion and we both had a good laugh when he found out that I wanted folic acid and iron.

But for many women the choice about whether or not to carry a pregnancy to term is no laughing matter. I remember a high school classmate who was spirited off to the Bahamas for an illegal abortion in the early 1960s. An outgoing, cheerful girl before she left, she returned sad and morose. Her parents were angry, the boy who had contributed his seed long gone, and her hormones were in an uproar. Furthermore, "Annie" was grieving for a child she would never know—and thirty years ago it had somehow escaped the mass mind that a woman might grieve an aborted child just as she would grieve a miscarriage.

The emergence of the family as we now know it is intimately connected to issues of birth control and abortion. Before this century lasting partnerships between men and women were relatively rare because women so frequently died in childbirth, or at an early age because of the cumulative physical and emotional stress of birthing and caring for huge families. Gradually, women began to limit family size through sexual abstinence, the poorly effective rhythm method, and illegal abortion. In her valuable book, *What Every American Should Know about Women's History*, Christine Lunardini summarizes statistics about changing family size, "In 1800, there were 7 children per woman in the United States. In 1900 there were only 3.5, and by 1940 just over 2."

The first American book on birth control was published by Robert Owen in 1830. Entitled *Moral Physiology*, it offered advice on birth control along with the philosophy that fewer, better-educated children would make a stronger country. This was exactly the argument that had brought Julia to Bangladesh, where women still mother enormous broods, often dying young from complications of childbirth, desperate attempts at abortion, or plain old exhaustion that depletes their immune systems and leaves them prey to infectious disease, ultimately orphaning their children.

Owen's belief that birth control was a woman's prerogative, and an important way to strengthen the family and society, was not widely supported in nineteenth-century America. It wasn't until three quarters of a century after Owen's book was published that Margaret Sanger and her sister, Ethel Byrne, opened a birth control clinic in Brooklyn, New York, in the fall of 1916. The sisters were motivated by their own mother's early death after having borne eleven children in rapid succession, and knew that for a woman to survive to nurture her offspring, she needed to know how to limit family size. But after only ten days, Sanger and Byrne were arrested for violating the infamous Comstock Law, and their clinic was shut down.

The Comstock Law, which Sanger ran afoul of repeatedly in attempting to disseminate information by mail or in person, dealt with obscenity. Anything pertaining to sex fell under the rubric of this puritanical law until it was finally altered by the federal courts in 1938, after which Sanger opened a chain of over three hundred birth control clinics across the country. The American Birth Control League that she founded eventually began to speak of family planning rather than birth control and evolved into the Planned Parenthood Association in 1942. Half a century later, emotions still run high over birth control, and especially abortion.

While abortion can be a difficult choice for women to make, almost half of all women do make it, three fifths of whom have their first abortion before they are twenty-one. What are the psychological effects? Psychologist Samuel Janus and obstetrician/gynecologist Cynthia Janus undertook a national survey of 4,510 women representing a cross-section of socioeconomic and religious groups. They found that about half of all women who had aborted felt relief while half reported guilt, regret, or sadness. When they investigated how women's religious beliefs affected their views about abortion, 55 percent of the very religious agreed strongly that abortion was murder, yet 18 percent of these religious women reported having had one, a choice that must have been particularly heartrending.

When a person is placed in a position where she feels compelled to act out of accord with strong beliefs, severe stress generally results. During the 1980s when I directed a mind/body clinic at Boston's Beth Israel Hospital, many women with stress-related disorders came to learn about emotional resiliency, stress hardiness, and relaxation. One of the most important things we did together was to revisit and heal unfinished business from the past—those regrets and resentments that were holding mind and body hostage. Some of the most poignant regrets that highly religious women spoke of were indeed centered on abortions. Andrea, for example, was a beautiful blond woman who was a cradle Catholic. Relying on the rhythm method, since the Church forbade other means of birth control, she and her college beau conceived a child. When you think about the wide range of cues that can affect female hormones—from smell to voice tone, from a man's place in the social hierarchy to whether he reads poetry or sends flowers—it's no wonder that the rhythm method of birth control so often fails. When the instinctual circuitry of the brain gets the message that a genetic match made in heaven is possible, an egg may pop out at a most unpropitious moment for the unsuspecting. Pheromones, for example, bind to receptors in the hypothalamus which, in turn, trigger the release of a tiny protein with the daunting designation GnRH, which stands for gonadotropin releasing hormone. Its role is to signal the pituitary gland to release follicular stimulating hormone (FSH) to coax the ovary into releasing an egg in response to the instinctually compelling charms of the would-be suitor.

Andrea's nineteen-year-old beau was ready for sex, but not for fatherhood. When they became another statistic in rhythm method failure, the young couple panicked. To have the child would have been a great stigma for them and their families, and would have meant the end of their education. With terrible remorse, Andrea had an abortion. No amount of prayer, confession, or acts of contrition could set her mind at ease. Ten years after the abortion, Andrea had chronic stomach pains and nausea. Married for four years, she was unable to conceive a child and fervently believed that she was being punished for her sins.

We had known one another for nearly a year before Andrea finally unburdened her heart. Having heard many stories of abortions, I knew that for some women it was hard to move on and complete their grieving without a powerful ritual to help transform the old wound into a new strength. We used meditation to construct a ritual in which Andrea could contact the soul of the baby she had aborted. She closed her eyes and relaxed deeply by focusing on the gentle rise of her body on the inhalation, and its relaxation on the exhalation. I asked her to imagine a sacred grove, a place filled with wisdom and light—a light that emanated wisdom, compassion, and forgiveness. She was able to feel that light washing through her body, carrying away guilt and confusion, revealing the pure light of love that was in her own heart. I then suggested that she allow her heart light to expand, filling her entire body and radiating out into the sacred grove, where she could then meet the soul of her unborn child.

Andrea's face filled with awe and radiance, then gentle tears began to run down her cheeks. "He's here," she whispered, "in the grove. He says that he is so glad I have come, so happy that I am finally ready to receive the gift he came to give me." In hushed tones, half in this world and half in another, Andrea narrated their communion. Raphael, the name by which the soul of her aborted child called himself, said that he was one of her guardian angels. He assured her that human beings grow by making difficult choices, and in the process, becoming more self-aware and more loving. He told her that he not only understood her choice to abort, but had been assigned to her at the beginning of her pregnancy precisely because of the likelihood that she would do so and would be in need of guidance and healing. Hence his name. In Hebrew, Raphael means "healer of God."

When Andrea asked Raphael what he would have done if she had carried the pregnancy through, he smiled and said that he would have taken birth in human form, guiding and loving her first as a child and then as an adult. He would always be with her in any case, he promised, ever available for help. Raphael told her that the most important lesson she had to learn was self-forgiveness. She had repented her actions—which means thinking them through and taking responsibility for them—and only forgiveness was required to complete the process.

I am always awed when I witness a healing like Andrea's. You might wonder if her communication with Raphael was "real" or whether it was a wishful fantasy of her mind. She asked the same question. I responded in the words of the Jesus she loved, "By their fruits ye shall know them." The fruits of the communion ritual with Raphael were many. Andrea's stomach pains disappeared and three months later she became pregnant. I have no doubt that the forgiveness she learned to extend to herself not only relieved her stress and made the pregnancy possible, but has helped make her a particularly caring and nurturing mother.

Abortion is an emotional issue—and because of the mind/body connection it can also be a physical one. The guilt and grief that some women suffer may, as in Andrea's case, even hinder their ability to conceive another child. Remember that the secretion of FSH and luteinizing hormone (LH) from the pituitary gland are, in turn, dependent on the release of GnRH from the hypothalamus which is, in turn, affected by emotional and physical stress. The simple stress of traveling, for example, often causes women to skip periods and may contribute to what are called anovulatory cycles in which the period comes, but no egg is released. Physical stress such as poor nutrition or too much exercise can result in similar upheavals of reproductive rhythm, as can any kind of serious emotional stress.

GIVING BIRTH: BIOLOGY VERSUS TECHNOLOGY

Julia was twenty-seven, a social worker in an obstetrical unit at a Boston hospital, when she conceived her first child. The average American woman becomes a mother at the age of twenty-six. Many of us are not "average" and become mothers earlier, later, or not at all. But for those of us who do birth babies, an entire industry exists that has medicalized a natural process that our bodies have been elegantly designed to perform. On the one hand this intervention often interferes with biological events that proceed more smoothly on their own. On the other hand it sometimes saves the lives of mother, child, or both. As with most things, knowledge of our bodies and our choices is critical in making the most of the birth process. And compared to women in previous centuries, we're lucky to have such a wide range of choices.

For many years the Church prohibited alleviating the pain of child-birth since that travail was thought to be woman's just due—punishment for Eve's sin in the garden. In *Of Woman Born*, feminist poet and writer Adrienne Rich cites the example of Agnes Simpson, a midwife who was burned at the stake in 1591 for using opium to relieve labor pains. Since the Church forbade dissection, medicine in Christian lands—as opposed to Middle Eastern countries where both Islamic and Jewish physicians were relatively well trained in anatomy—remained primitive.

Midwives, however, had intimate knowledge of the female anatomy, moon cycles, and the birth process. Unfortunately, they were widely feared by the male Church hierarchy for their knowledge of herbs that could prevent conception or lead to abortion, and for their ability to alleviate the pain of childbirth. Like Agnes Simpson, many midwives were burned at the stake either because they were accused of being witches, or for practicing medicine without a license. Since one had to attend medical school to be licensed, and only men were admitted to such schools, midwives had to practice their healing arts in secret or risk death. During the Middle Ages many women preferred to birth their babies unassisted if midwives were unavailable since delivery at the hands of unskilled physicians was risky business.

In the late sixteenth century the birthing process took a dramatic turn. A family of physicians by the name of Chamberlain invented the obstetrical forceps and developed a widespread reputation for success-fully aiding complicated births. Although the family kept their instrument to themselves for two generations, by 1773 the secret was out. While the ability to pull a baby free was a great boon for difficult labors and breech births, it soon fell into common use for all labors. By this time the Inquisition with its rash of witch burnings had ceased and midwives were once again in practice. They pointed out, quite rightly, that forceps were an intervention that, when used unnecessarily, endangered both mother and child.

The competition between midwives and physicians was decided in favor of the former when a two-century long plague of childbed fever decimated European mothers delivered by physicians beginning in the seventeenth century. Childbed, or puerperal, fever, was caused by bacterial sepsis. Physicians would dissect corpses, attend to wounds, do surgery, and then deliver babies with their unwashed hands. Germs traveled directly through the abraded lining of the uterus to the blood, and a painful death followed for an infected mother a few days later. Adrienne Rich wrote that in the French province of Lombardy during one year, not a single woman survived childbirth in the local hospital. Although midwives were also ignorant of the relation between germs and disease, the average home was much cleaner than the hospitals, and midwives were not dissecting corpses or attending wounds prior to assisting the laboring woman.

Considering the long, dark history of birthing, today's mother has better choices. She can bring her child into the world at home, in a typical hospital setting, or in a hospital with a birthing center where both labor and delivery occur in a homelike room. Nonetheless, the birth process has become overly technical, and the ancient debate between midwives and physicians about the degree of intervention required in a normal birth is as relevant now as it was in the 1700s. Julia and Roger got caught up in this same debate. Julia wanted to deliver her baby at home with Roger's assistance, or with a midwife. Roger, on the other hand, was afraid of possible complications and felt that he could never forgive himself if anything happened to Julia or their child. In the end they made a compromise, and Julia delivered their daughter, Amanda, in a hospital "home-birth" room with the assistance of a midwife.

When Justin, my firstborn, arrived in 1969 there were not yet any home-birth centers in hospitals. Natural childbirth had just begun to replace the older practices of anesthetizing the mother with a combination of drugs called "twilight sleep" that sometimes compromised the vital functions of the baby. I took Lamaze breathing classes and was ready for so-called natural childbirth. I arrived at the hospital in the middle of a heavy snowstorm in February, not because I was in labor, but because strong Braxton-Hicks contractions had gone on for about twelve hours and the doctor was afraid that if labor started I might not be able to get to the hospital through the storm.

Even though labor had not technically begun, my cervix was dilated to about five centimeters, an excellent start. But rather than let things proceed naturally, the doctor gave me a shot of pitocin (a pituitary hormone that initiates labor) to speed things along, estimating that the baby might come in ten to twelve hours. I went right into heavy labor and the amniotic membranes were ruptured to expedite the process further. Within two hours I felt the urge to push. The nurse, who didn't bother to check on the degree of dilation, just assumed that it was too early. But the body cannot be denied. I pushed secretly, simply because the pain disappeared and a wonderful sense of opening and relief accompanied it. After four or five pushes I became aware of pressure between my legs.

The baby was about to make his debut in the labor room bed! And what would have been wrong with that? I called the nurse, who panicked at the sight of Justin's crowning and rushed me to the delivery room screaming, "Pant, pant! Don't push!" Fear immediately interrupted my labor and I had no further need to push. The natural flow had been interrupted. In the delivery room I was given saddle block anesthesia, an episiotomy, and Justin was pulled out with forceps. His eyes were treated with silver nitrate, a standard practice I couldn't stop, and he was wrapped and taken away to the nursery. It was several hours before I saw him again. At that point he seemed to belong to the nurse and I felt like an interloper. To this day I wish that I'd kept my mouth shut and birthed him in the bed. We were doing just fine on our own without a painful technological finale to what had been a relatively painless, intimate, and natural birth. Experiences like mine are still the norm in hospitals, where normal births are often complicated even further by the use of fetal monitoring equipment, all in the name of "natural childbirth."

THE BIOLOGY OF MOTHERHOOD: INFATUATION AND THE NEWBORN

Maternal behavior begins long before birth. Rats begin to construct nests and women clean the house and reorganize their closets. The night before going into labor with Amanda, Julia was seized with an undeniable desire to stand on a rickety stepladder and scrub the kitchen ceiling. For a woman who closely resembled an artichoke on legs even to tilt her head back and look at the ceiling was a feat. Actually to restore it to a pristine white perfection was a miracle. Hormones, once again, are the mediators of such strange miracles.

As the body gears up to nourish a growing baby, levels of estrogen and progesterone both increase. Progesterone causes the uterine lining to thicken with blood vessels and eventually form a placenta, or life-support system, that delivers nutrients to the baby and carries off wastes. The presence of the fetus stimulates the placenta to release human placental lactogen (HPL) which causes the glandular tissue in the breasts to increase in preparation for making milk. The wonderful cascade of biological changes that allow a mother to nourish her baby continue at birth when the pituitary gland begins to secrete large quantities of the hormone prolactin which coaxes the prepared breasts to begin milk production. And both HPL and prolactin act directly on the hypothalamus, stimulating maternal behavior that goes far beyond nesting. Like a bear protecting her cubs, most human mothers will risk life and limb to protect their offspring. Indeed, the urge to protect life in all its forms is one of the most remarkable gifts of women.

At birth, another hormone made in the hypothalamus, oxytocin, comes into play. It not only stimulates the uterus to contract when released during labor, but also causes uterine contractions when secreted in response to nursing. As the uterus contracts, blood vessels are closed off, lessening the chance for hemorrhage. It also stimulates milk "letdown," or in the first few days after birth, the letdown of colostrum (a nutrient fluid made by the glandular tissue of the breast before milk production begins). Some women who are stressed, for example, have milk in their breasts but can't let it down into the ducts where it is available for nursing because stress inhibits the release of oxytocin. This is why some women can only nurse in the privacy of their homes, but not in strange places and some can nurse quite well until their mother-in-law arrives for a visit.

The nerve cells that secrete oxytocin into the bloodstream also send axons to other areas of the brain and spinal cord. Messages from these axons create mild, pleasant sexual arousal—another trick of nature to ensure that we will enjoy nursing our babies. Toward the end of pregnancy there are specific changes in two groups of cells located within the hypothalamus, called the supraoptic nucleus (SON) and the paraventricular nucleus (PVN), which secrete oxytocin. Before the mother gives birth, the neurons within these nuclei are separated from one another by glial cells. A few hours after birth, the "veil" of glial cells moves away, bringing the oxytocin-secreting cells into direct connection with one another. This connection activates the cells and stimulates oxytocin release. Simultaneously we bond with our newborn, the very sight, sound, and smell of the child releasing oxytocin, which creates feelings of warmth, contentment, and arousal. Once again, biology has created infatuation to make sure that we will dote on our babies.

Emotionally healthy mothers like Julia are as unconditionally loving toward their newborns as they are toward potential mates in the infatuation phase of courtship. Once again, love is blind. Julia gets that adoring look in her eyes as she repeatedly shows off birth pictures of red, wrinkled Amanda to anyone who will look. Maternal love at first sight is another biological gift for if it did not occur the burdens of caring for a helpless infant might be overwhelming. When Julia first brought little Amanda home from the hospital, she was tired and overwhelmed with caring for the baby's needs. Fortunately, Grandma Sylvia came to help for the first few days, but even so Julia had to breast-feed the wakeful Amanda nearly every two hours, interrupting her own sleep. Fortunately, Julia was duly infatuated with her little bundle and performed the superhuman feats of mothering with an energy that is similar to that produced by PEA in lovers.

What about mothers who for one reason or another are unable or choose not to breast-feed their infants. Do we bond with bottle-fed babies in the same way? We do bond, of course, although the biological and behavioral pathways are likely to be different. Fortunately, hormones are not the only mediator of maternal behavior. A female rat who has never had pups will begin to act maternally after several days of contact with another mother's offspring. In the case of humans, there are even documented cases of adoptive mothers who eventually produce milk and nurse their babies.

When nursing mothers wean their young, the veil of glial cells between the oxytocin-producing neurons in the hypothalamus moves back into place. The baby is no longer a source of comfort and arousal in the same sense that it was before, and neither is it so helpless. Her smiles and laughter have created another kind of bonding. Just as we generally move out of infatuation into attachment and then on to true love with our mates, so the progression proceeds with our babies if we are emotionally healthy enough to be good mothers.

THE BIO-PSYCHO-SPIRITUAL GIFTS OF RELATING TO MATES AND CHILDREN

As we have seen, a woman's biology is specially crafted to produce pleasure, excitement, and joy for her in the ancient dance of relationship when the smell, sight, and touch of her potential beloved excite the pathways between the rhinencephalon and limbic system that release the relational molecule called PEA. The resultant biochemically sustained infatuation gives rise to strong spiritual experiences of interconnectedness and deep communion. But a short-lived biochemical high, unfortunately, does not always set the stage for true love. It is like a temporary state of grace on which an authentic, intimate relationship must then be built.

The exquisite psychobiological feedback loop that evolved to ensure infatuation with genetically suitable mates has an important cognitive, or thinking, component built in through our neocortex. We can reflect on the relational qualities of our possible mate, and ideally overcome the chemical euphoria of attraction if our potential partner is psychologically unsuitable. We ask ourselves: Is he capable of real intimacy, of sharing his feelings and acknowledging mine? Can I continue to find my true self, a self-in-relation with him? Will we be able to encourage and bring out the best in one another? Do we share common values? Will he be able to have a loving relationship with any children we might have? If the answer to most of these questions is no, when our temporary biochemical infatuation dissipates, lasting attachment is unlikely to occur because the psychospiritual side of the feedback loop that encourages mutual development is lacking.

But what happens when a woman is not mature enough to ask the questions of relationship authenticity? Since the development of a strong sense of self-in-relation occurs for women in adolescence, and in the best case begins to mature only in her early twenties, it is little wonder that most teen marriages fail. The biological circuits of infatuation were in place, but the psychospiritual counterparts were still maturing, making it more difficult to choose an emotionally healthy partner. A woman who has not yet resolved the developmental dilemma, "How can I get my own needs met without being selfish toward others?" may give herself away to a man, honoring his opinions, needs, and desires without considering her own. The result is that she loses herself in the relationship rather than growing through it. Another common mistake that women who have not resolved the dilemma make is that they see a man's problems, but believe that they can change him, rescue him, or reform him. "If I only love him enough," she thinks, "he'll change." But he usually doesn't. These types of problems reflect the fact that the peak time for divorce is in the midtwenties, when early relationship misjudgments come home to roost.

The psychobiological gifts of womanhood extend to relationships with our infants. When the veil of glial cells between oxytocin-producing cells in the hypothalamus breaks down in the process of giving birth, so does the boundary between ourself and our child. The oneness we feel not only allows milk to be let down for nursing, but also results in a state of communion similar to the one that we first felt toward our mate. Once again, however, a psychospiritual feedback loop must be in place so that the biological predilection for bonding can proceed to mutually enhancing relationship. If a mother has not come into her own sense of self, her ability to relate to her child after the initial state of union dissipates is also limited. The trend toward having children later in life is important in this regard, because the more psychologically mature the mother is, the more the child will have an opportunity for optimal development.

All through childhood and adolescence, a girl has been immersed in the relational world, preparing for her special role in sustaining the network of interdependent connectedness between herself and others, and between people and nature. The quality of the intense relationships that begin to emerge in our twenties is both a testimony to what we may have already learned, and a warning about what things may not yet have been mastered. The emergent spirituality of relationship is not a developmental stage with a distinct beginning and end, but a lifelong path whose markers are happiness, creativity, compassion, and a satisfying sense of mutual growth. The fact that our brain circuits are plastic and changeable means that we can profit from emotional feedback and change our course, thoughts, and behavior when the satisfaction inherent in relationality is not present.

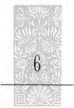

AGES 28–35: THE AGE 30 TRANSITION

NEW REALITIES, NEW PLANS

Julia's best friend, Liza, a thirty-two-year-old hospital administrator, has been married to her husband, Rob, for six years. Like many career-oriented women, she wanted to devote herself to climbing the corporate ladder before thinking about having a family. During her twenties she felt in charge of her life, moving ahead, learning new job skills, and finally meeting and marrying a man she felt would be her life partner. Now her carefully tailored plan is falling apart at the seams. Convinced that the only requirement for advancement was doing a good job, Liza has awakened to the reality that most corporate structures are pyramidal. With every step up the ladder the rungs become shorter and fewer jobs are available. Those that are available become the focus of intense competition and political wrangling that she finds unfair, inhumane, and distasteful.

Passed over for promotion when a male colleague made false insinuations about her dependence on other members of the team for her creative ideas, she became disheartened. Didn't people work best when they pooled their ideas and brainstormed? Cooperation made intellectual and emotional sense, but it was not the politically correct way to operate in her competitive corporate structure. The Lone Ranger types were obviously the ones who jockeyed their way ahead, often at the expense of others. Liza wonders if she spent so much time, effort, and money getting an MBA for nothing. The way that the hospital operates feels out of synch with her values, and furthermore she feels stalled in a job, only two notches above entry level, in which she endlessly reviews quality control issues for the hospital's risk management team.

Liza entered hospital administration with the hope that she could make a difference, that she could help humanize the health-care system. Now she feels like an assembly line worker destined to install the same widget over and over, with little hope for advancement. Coupled with her rude career awakening, the fact that she has been trying to get pregnant for two and a half years without success has left her feeling almost desperate. Whatever happened, she wonders, to the raven-haired whiz kid, as she was called in graduate school? Only a few years later, nothing seems to be going the way she planned.

THE AGE 30 TRANSITION

The late Yale psychologist Daniel J. Levinson, who was widely hailed for his research on the male life cycle that was the basis for his 1978 best-seller, *The Seasons of a Man's Life*, did a similar study of the female life cycle that centered on in-depth interviews with forty-five women, focusing on the years between their late teens and midforties. He makes the point that in early and middle adulthood the process of adolescing, or growing up, coexists with the process of senescing, or growing down, periods when our life structures go into decline. The life structure is defined as a boundary between ourselves and the external world that functions as a framework for occupational and family relationships. It is composed of our hopes and dreams, values and talents. How will we fit into the world? What is important to us? What will make us happy?

The period that spans the late teens to midforties, in Levinson's model, is one of building the life structure for our young adulthood. The early thirties are what he calls a "structure-changing or transitional period [that] terminates the existing life structure and creates the possibility for a new one." Experiences like Liza's, during which her early dream of making a difference in the health-care system, along with her hope of becoming a mother, are "senescing," are typical of women in her part of the life cycle. She has followed her dream and ended up in territory that is not to her liking, and is now engaged in a reappraisal of her situation that will lead to a new cycle of adolescing, a further evolution. The major task involved in the age thirty transition, which Levinson found to span the years between twenty-eight and thirty-two, is the exploration of new possibilities and the finishing up of old business that may be getting in the way of a woman's continued growth.

Inherent in reevaluating what Levinson calls our "necessarily flawed" early life structures (after all, what adolescent can possibly foresee the many circuitous routes of her life when she makes initial plans to enter the adult world?), are nagging questions about how to combine work and family, whether to combine work and family, and whether early marriage partnerships are working out. These questions may be further confounded by the stress of infertility. Like Liza, many women in their thirties want to be mothers but either cannot conceive or have trouble carrying the pregnancy to term. Will they persevere in trying to conceive or alter their life plan? Central to a woman's age thirty transition is the question, "What do I really want?"

What Does a Woman Want?

Wellesley College psychologists Grace Baruch and Rosalind Barnett, in collaboration with Boston University journalism professor Caryl Rivers, published a landmark study of women, family, work and love in 1983. It is called the Lifeprints Study. They were trying to answer a question that Freud once voiced in abject frustration, "What does a woman want?" Among the strong points of the study were the questions they asked about the rewards and pleasures in women's lives.

Prior to the 1960s a woman was supposed to want to stay home and live the life of the "pampered" housewife, learning the art of manipulating her husband into supplying her with the latest time-saving conveniences. The problem, of course, was cutting all women out of the same piece of cloth. Like men, we have different needs and wants. Some women bloom in the role of homemaker, others fade. Some of us fulfill our urge to mother through bearing children, others through nourishing siblings, friends, parents, or ideas. There is no one life story that fits us all. Every woman who works and mothers is not destined for burnout, nor is a woman who stays home and mothers her children necessarily unable to resume her career at thirty-five or forty.

Their research involved a random sample of three hundred Massachusetts women between thirty-five and fifty-five. The average educational level was high—fourteen years—or two years past high school. Theirs was an unusually well educated group, and like this book, likely to be more resonant with the experience of white middle- and upper-class women than women of color and those at low socioeconomic levels. Just to give you some perspective, 1991 statistics revealed that only two in five American women twenty-five years of age and over had completed high school; only one in five had completed college. These statistics, by the way, are for white women. Black and Hispanic women are statistically less likely to complete college, while women of Asian descent are more likely than whites to get a college degree.

The Lifeprints Study is fascinating because it documents the major shift that has occurred in women's life patterns. The authors write, "When the women in our study were growing up, working women were the 'deviant' group, and they often felt isolated and stigmatized. Today, however, it is the homemakers in our sample who feel alone and misunderstood by those around them, while working women are experiencing a newfound sense of support. These trends are not likely to be reversed in the years ahead: the lives of the women in our sample are therefore highly relevant to women who are now in their twenties or early thirties." The authors were correct. The trends they speak of have continued to strengthen over the two decades since their study was published.

The women in their research sample were divided into six groups: never married, employed; married without children, employed; married with children, employed; divorced with children, employed; married with children, at home; and married without children, at home. In a scale called Mastery, which measures self-esteem and confidence, working women were all in or near the top half, scoring much higher on average than homemakers. The women lowest on the Mastery scale were married women without children who stayed at home. Divorced women, by the way, topped the Mastery scale. This dovetails with other research that demonstrates the advantages of learning to cope with difficult situations and remaking your life after a major crisis. The groups that scored highest on Pleasure were married women with children who stayed home, and married women with children who worked. The groups scoring lowest on Pleasure were married women without children who stayed home, unmarried women at work, and divorced mothers who worked.

The authors were fascinated to discover the high well-being (the combination of Mastery and Pleasure) of "the busiest women in our study, the employed, married women with children." My mother might have been surprised with the Lifeprints data, but I am not. Although I'm prone to do my share of bitching and groaning about being so busy even now, when the children are out on their own, I look back at my mother's life with poignant memories of her unhappiness. The Lifeprints Study would have found my brilliant, beautiful mother low in both Mastery and Pleasure. But in her time and social class, she had little choice other than to remain at home being a homemaker at first without children, then with children, and once again without children after we had grown up.

I look back both with amusement (her impassioned pleas for me to act stupid so that I wouldn't frighten men away, for example, were actually funny to both of us) and a certain sadness at her heartfelt attempts to raise me in the image of Betty Friedan's feminine mystique. But after all, only a single generation ago that was the gold standard for women—a standard measured by motherhood. Not surprisingly, my mother's two greatest fears for me centered on having children. While I was a teenager, her most terrible fantasy was that I might get pregnant before marriage. Later, her fear was that I might choose career over children. And a life without children was incomprehensible to her.

Does Mothering Require Children?

The authors of the Lifeprints Study document how emotion laden the issue of whether or not to have children is to the modern woman. Indeed, it is a critical question for career women engaged in the age thirty transition, and the reassessment of their life structure that comes at this time. In my mother's generation, the question rarely arose since it was just assumed that married women who were healthy would have children. It was both our biological destiny and the act that was assumed to lead to psychological and spiritual fulfillment. The question of motherhood is often debated in terms of two extremes: the idea that women without children will feel empty and unfulfilled versus the idea that women with children have signed up for a life of "indentured servitude."

In reality, the question of whether or not to mother is neither black or white, but is shaded by the quality of all our other relationships, goals, and natural predilections. The simple idea that women must mother to feel whole, and that motherhood is the ultimate source of fulfillment, is refuted not only by the data of the Lifeprints researchers, but by a poll they cite of Ann Landers's readers. When she asked mothers if they would choose to repeat the experience, an incredible 70 percent said no, reflecting the fact that motherhood has its inevitable share of conflicts and is not a one-way ticket to heaven.

According to the Lifeprints data, being childless had no particular influence on either Mastery or Pleasure unless a woman who wanted children was unable to resolve not having them. Interestingly, women turn out to be more hesitant about having children than do men; they are more realistic about the difficulties and sacrifices that are involved. The decision whether or not to have children involves weighing a tremendous number of factors—emotional, economic, and physical. Both motherhood and the decision not to mother have their own benefits and liabilities.

While a child is inherent to the traditional idea of motherhood, many of the 20 percent of women who are childless have found other ways to mother. One can mother godchildren, siblings, and parents; ideas, communities, and projects; plants, animals, and the natural world. Six of my closest women friends are childless; three by choice and three by circumstance. All of them are reconciled to their child-lessness and lead full and interesting lives. Three of these women and I gathered one evening to talk about the different ways that childless women mother. One is a married obstetrician/gynecologist who chose not to have children, but has helped birth hundreds of babies. She is one of the most nurturing people I know, dedicated to teaching women how to care for themselves, plan for their families (which includes tak-ing the necessary steps not to have children when this is their choice), and bring healthy babies into the world. Mentoring other physicians has been an important form of mothering for her. And without the stress of children, her marriage has been a particularly close and sup-portive experience. Another friend is an unmarried nurse, researcher, and professor, the oldest of five children. Although technically child-less, she mothered all her siblings including a younger brother who was thirteen years her junior. Once again, she mentioned the many men and women that she has mentored during her career as a form of moth-ering. A third unmarried friend is a hospice worker and healer who nurtures the spirits of those facing death, and their families. In a very real sense she helps people give birth to their souls when their time on earth is complete. In a world that is already overpopulated, she believes that her choice not to bear children is also a way to nurture a planet whose resources have been so badly depleted.

We are living in a time when women have a multitude of choices about family and career. But the ancient archetype of the Great Mother has never been more important than it is today. Through our growing awareness and power, women both with and without children are helping to birth a new world. Our ability to connect, to nurture, and to make decisions based on present and future needs rather than past conventions are the hope of this planet and the children who col-lectively belong to us all.

THE CHALLENGE OF INFERTILITY

But what about the woman, like Liza, who wants to mother a biologi-cal child and finds that she and her husband can't seem to conceive? Psychologist Alice D. Domar, director of the Women's Health Programs at the Mind/Body Institute at the New England Deaconess Hospital, Harvard Medical School, found that women trying unsuccessfully to become pregnant have stress levels, in terms of anxiety and depression, equivalent to women with cancer, HIV, and heart disease. Conception can become the main focus of their lives, putting them on a roller-coaster ride that ends with dashed hopes once a month when their periods arrive. Tracking ovulation can take all the fun and spontaneity out of sex, and marital disruption is common.

Statistically one in six couples, or 15 percent of those who want children, face infertility. Many women in such couples are in their thirties. In about 40 percent of these cases the problem originates with the man, in 60 percent with the woman. There has been increasing publicity about decreasing sperm counts in many different countries, both in men and in animals like alligators who live in the pesticide-laden waters of the Florida Everglades. Although research is not yet conclusive, there is mounting evidence that pesticides containing molecules with estrogenlike activity (xenoestrogens) affect the male reproductive system leading to undescended testicles, micropenises, and lower sperm counts. They may also cause reproductive difficulties in women and are being investigated as a possible cause of breast cancer. About 20 percent of all infertility is attributed to unknown causes; there are no physical abnormalities either in the man or the woman sufficient to explain the problem.

Gynecologist Christiane Northrup ascribes unexplained infertility to five causes: irregular ovulation, fallopian tubes scarred by infection or IUDs, immunological problems in which women make antibodies against the sperm of their mate, endometriosis, and stress. The latter two problems are prevalent enough to take a closer look. Endometriosis is a condition in which the kinds of cells that line the uterus (endometrial cells) are found outside of the uterus, usually in the peritoneal (pelvic) cavity where they may be growing on the ovaries, the fallopian tubes, the intestines or the body wall. At times they may migrate as far away as the lungs. These cells respond to hormones just the way they do in the uterus, multiplying during the first half of the menstrual cycle, attracting a rich blood supply during the latter half of the cycle, and then finally shedding their upper layers in a menstrual flow. These cyclic changes and releases of blood can cause chronic pain, bloating, severe menstrual cramps, heavy periods, and pain during intercourse, as well as leaving scars on the ovaries and fallopian tubes that may lead to infertility. This condition is found primarily in menstruating women between the ages of twenty and forty-five, and its peak incidence is in the thirties.

The cause of endometriosis is unclear, although the most prevalent theory is that all women push some endometrial cells out through the fallopian tubes when the uterus spasms during their period, a process called retrograde menstruation. The question that has not yet been answered is why these cells are simply resorbed by some women, while they implant and grow in others. One theory is that women with compromised immune function are unable to halt the spread of this tissue into a location where it would not normally grow. The definitive diagnosis of endometriosis can only be made by inserting a small, lighted tube called a laparoscope into the abdomen, and actually looking for islands of endometrial cells or the scars they have left. Oddly, some women with large amounts of endometriosis suffer few symptoms, while others with fewer patches of wayward cells, suffer more.

The old psychosomatic theory of endometriosis cast it as the career women's disease, a problem that was believed to afflict women who were outgoing, competitive, and who delayed childbearing. Since estrogen stimulates the growth of the endometrial implants, some researchers do believe that pregnancy helps halt the progression of the disease since it affords some hiatus from cyclical hormonal fluctuations. However, the condition is clearly the result of more than either career stress or lack of pregnancy. Women whose mothers or sisters have endometriosis are at an elevated risk, indicating a genetic predisposition. Caucasians are much more prone than blacks, women with chronic infections and other stresses to the immune system are at increased risk, as are those who use estrogen-dominant birth control pills or who are overweight.

The medical treatment of endometriosis may involve surgery to remove the endometrial implants and reduce scar tissue, or hormonal therapy including drugs that induce a temporary state of menopause to decrease circulating levels of estrogen. After several months the drugs are discontinued, and symptoms may be relieved. Physician Susan Lark has had great success in helping women to decrease symptoms in a natural, noninvasive way with a program of symptom monitoring, stress reduction, gentle yoga-type stretches, meditation and guided imagery, and diet. She specifically suggests eliminating or severely restricting the intake of dairy products because they are rich in arachidonic acid, a precursor to F2 alpha prostaglandins, which increase muscle spasms and can worsen pelvic pain and cramping. The high fat content of dairy foods also favors excess estrogen production, which in women who eat a diet high in animal fats can be twice the amount of estrogen in that of vegetarians eating a low-fat, high-fiber diet.

Stress may not only be a factor in endometriosis, which in itself can lead to infertility, it may also be a cause of infertility. The question of whether stress causes infertility or infertility creates stress has been hotly debated with no scientific resolution. But Dr. Domar's research proves unequivocally that women coping with infertility are highly stressed whatever the cause; they are twice as likely to be depressed as women going to the gynecologist for routine checkups, and have stress levels similar to women with serious illness. Stress can inhibit ovulation as well as cause spasms of the fallopian tubes that may hinder the sperm from reaching the egg.

A question that several researchers have asked is whether stress reduction can aid in conception. Dr. Domar, whom I had the pleasure to supervise during her early clinical training in mind/body medicine, is a pioneer in this regard. In 1978 she developed a ten-week group program (women attend one two-hour session each week) for women with unexplained infertility. Based on coping-skills training, learning to shift from the stress response to the relaxation response, guided imagery, gentle yoga stretching, good nutrition, education in topics pertinent to fertility, and support from other women in the group, the program has an excellent track record in reducing women's stress. The emphasis is on shifting the focus of life away from conceiving a baby to living a creative, fulfilling life in other regards, as described in the excellent book she coauthored with science writer Henry Dreher, *Healing Mind, Healthy Woman.*

When women ask Dr. Domar what the success rate of her program is, she smiles and replies that it is 98 percent, since almost all the women who complete it have significant reductions in anxiety, anger, and depression, and an increase in vitality and well-being. Single-minded in pursuit of pregnancy, these women are really asking what the conception rate is. Although the program is designed only to reduce stress, statistics compiled from the nearly three hundred women who completed the program and were available for follow-up indicated that 57 percent of them became pregnant within six months of completing the ten-week course, a very encouraging side effect of the stress-reduction program.

When a woman has put off into her thirties having children as Liza did, hoping to get her career on track before becoming a mother, her chances of infertility increase not only owing to stress, exposure to environmental toxins and possibly to endometriosis, but because her eggs themselves are aging. All the eggs that a woman ever produces are in her ovaries by the time she is born, so when she is thirty, her eggs are also thirty years old. Research indicates that those eggs begin to degenerate progressively over time, increasing not only the incidence of Down's syndrome children as the mother ages, but also increasing the chances of producing an infertile egg. A friend of mine who is an obstetrician/gynecologist counsels women who want children to do so as early in life as their situation will allow. This was the case for Julia, whose first child, Amanda, was born when she was twenty-seven, and whose second child, Benjamin, was born four years later.

COMPROMISE, BALANCE, AND REEVALUATION OF THE LIFE STRUCTURE

When Amanda was a bright, vocal child of three, Julia became pregnant for the second time. Like many young mothers who work, her world was already a delicate balancing act between six essential types of relationship; to her husband, her child, her self, her work, friends, and extended family. Each of these relationships, in turn, was affected by others such as Roger's relationship to Amanda and the rest of her family. Adding a new baby to the mix will introduce another level of richness and complexity over which Julia has less control than she might fantasize. At least when you marry you have some notion about the personality of your mate. Having kids, however, has been compared to the turn of a roulette wheel, and it has been argued that women generally score lower than men in well-being because they have primary responsibility for the children. As any mother knows, their problems are your problems and there are generally lots of them. Furthermore, the inability to prevent problems from arising and the fact that there are not always easy solutions is thought to make women feel vulnerable, inadequate, and incompetent, a rather big fly in the proverbial apple pie.

Julia went into labor with Benjamin three weeks early. As his lusty cries filled the birthing room, Julia and Roger both had the impression that Benjamin was furious. In the months that followed, he cried often and angrily, and like Julia herself as an infant, was colicky and hard to comfort. The delicate balance of familial and work relationships was seriously disrupted as attempts to comfort Benjamin took priority. Chaos prevailed in the household, and for the first time in her life, Julia wondered if she had bitten off more than she could chew.

In 1992, 60 percent of women with children under six were in Julia's position, combining work and mothering. The kind of work that a mother does, whether or not her husband is willing to take part in managing home and family, and whether she views her family or her career as the primary determinant of her life structure, has a great deal to do with the age thirty transition and the reevaluation of her life plan. Levinson's sample of forty-five women comprised two groups who articulated different life structures. Homemakers, while they may have worked at jobs outside the home for economic or other reasons, had clearly defined marriage and family as their most important concern as they set out to begin their adult lives. Their work, if any, was secondary to their primary role as homemaker. Career women, while many also had families, initially had an investment in building a life either in the traditionally male-dominated business or academic worlds that either took precedence over family matters, or existed in a co-equal, but often uneasy, balance.

Most of the women in Levinson's homemaker sample were employed in unskilled or semiskilled jobs like typing, sales, clerical work, or food service that allowed them to move in and out of the workforce in response to the needs of their families. Others were involved in predominantly female occupations like teaching, social work, or nursing, occupations that I certainly consider careers, even though these women defined their life structures as that of homemakers. Each woman was interviewed in depth, several times over a period of two to three months, yielding an average of three hundred pages of transcribed notes in which the woman told her life story to a sympathetic interviewer who elicited relevant information about what the most important things were to the woman, and how she saw her life unfolding from her late teens through her thirties, or some cases her forties. Levinson identified two internalized figures within women's psyches; the Traditional Homemaker Figure was one archetypal image, the Antitraditional Figure was its nemesis. The latter called women to greater independence, to seek more in life than managing home and family, and to financial self-sufficiency. The internal struggles between these two archetypes were like warring voices that goaded women into reconsidering their life structures, including work and marriage.

By the age thirty transition, women in the homemaker sample were reaching new balances between the warring archetypes. The three main shifts that the women made were: making family and occupation equally central components of their life; keeping homemaking central but reducing their involvement in family while taking on part-time or volunteer jobs that gave them a sense of competence and independence; and getting legally or psychologically divorced, in other words, distancing themselves from their husbands and functioning much like single mothers although the husband was still present in the household. In the years between twenty-eight and thirty-three, eight of the fifteen homemakers arrived at the conclusion that their marriages had failed. Four divorced legally, five psychologically. The women who chose to divorce legally, and to enter the world of single mothers, were not as well off financially. Each described a tremendous struggle in providing for her children, since child support from husbands was either insufficient or nonexistent. The women also described a sense of exhilaration, of new independence, and of finding themselves that speaks well of the resiliency of women who make difficult, but life-affirming choices to revamp their life structure no matter the perils and costs.

There were thirty women in Levinson's career woman sample; fifteen who worked in the corporate world and fifteen academics. All shared an initial life structure in which going to work or graduate school would allow her to become autonomous, independent, and successful so that when she finally married later in her twenties, she wouldn't be swallowed up in a traditional type of marriage where the needs of the woman are secondary to those of the man. Most of these women hoped that they could take some time off when their children were born, allowing their husbands to be the chief providers for a time, until they resumed their careers. Only about two thirds of the career women were married by the age thirty transition, in contrast to all of the women in the homemaker sample. During the period of reevaluation, nine of the twenty-one who were married got legally divorced, and two had divorced earlier in their twenties. For the seven career women who had never married, the age thirty transition served as a prod to find a suitable mate, since they felt that time to start a family was running short. And for the sixteen (more than 50 percent of the women) who were childless, either married or single, the specter of missing out on motherhood began to become a significant source of stress.

The great majority (90 percent) of the career women found themselves in a life situation somewhat similar to Liza's. They were in moderate or serious crisis mode, focusing on a particular problem. Many voiced Liza's dilemma: Should I stay in a job where I feel stalemated or move on? Others were caught on the horns of a love dilemma. Which is worse, to remain stuck in an empty marriage or endure both the hurt of ending the relationship and the risk that nothing better will come along? Some were bothered by problems concerning children. Like Julia, they were overwhelmed with the responsibilities of mothering. Or like Liza, they were overwhelmed by the fear that they would not be able to bear children. In all cases the crisis posed questions about how the woman wanted to live, forcing her to clarify her goals and values. This clarification led to another set of questions about what changes she would need to make in her life in order to pursue another plan.

Levinson writes, "By their late thirties most of these career women came to understand the illusory nature of the image of Superwoman, who could 'do it all' with grace and flair. Their image was more that of the Juggler, who kept many spheres in the air without dropping any or losing a step in the perpetual forward motion. While continually seeking balance, most women found it impossible to give anything like equal priority to the various components of their life structure." The women tended to end up putting occupation first and mothering second. Trailing far behind was marriage, and time for leisure and friends was nearly nonexistent. Nonetheless, Levinson's data corroborates conclusions from the Wellesley College Lifeprints Study. Even though their lives were hectic and exhausting, most of the career women were satisfied were their situations overall. Career women with children also realized that the years of peak juggling would be over when their children left home, affording a more peaceful, balanced life in the future.

THE GIFTS AND CHALLENGES OF YOUNG ADULTHOOD: THE STORY OF BLUEBEARD

Clarissa Pinkola Estés, a Jungian analyst, *cantadora* (keeper of the old stories in the Latina tradition), and poet, first heard this unique version of this classic story of young womanhood from her Hungarian aunt Kathé. She includes her own literary version and rich and provocative psychological commentary of the tale in her fine book *Women Who Run with the Wolves*. I am indebted to her for her permission to retell this story, and for the gateway she provides into understanding a crucial developmental task of young adulthood. The young heroine of Bluebeard, like all of us, must let go of the mask of sweet naïveté that corresponds to the archetype Levinson calls the Traditional Homemaker Figure. In facing the dark urges of the Antitraditional Figure that lurks beneath the mask, we find an authentic power that saves body and soul—the power to see, hear, and know what is real, rather than to live a constricted, artificial, fairy-tale existence. In short, we arrive at the age thirty transition and are seriously confronted with the need to wrest our power from old archetypes and step more fully into our evolving selves.

Bluebeard is a threatening man, his sinister nature marked by a strange blue cast to his beard. He courts three sisters simultaneously, but none are initially interested because they intuitively fear him. But one day he convinces the three young women and their mother to go on a horseback ride and picnic, which everyone enjoys. Nonetheless, the older two sisters remain frightened of him. The youngest one, however, begins to rationalize his strangeness and tell herself that perhaps his beard is not so blue after all. They marry and she takes up residence in his enormous castle of a hundred rooms. He leaves for a trip one day, entrusting her with a giant key ring and the instruction that she may enter any room except the one that the smallest key opens.

Her sisters arrive for a visit and they make a game of discovering which door the littlest key fits. When they open the door, the room is dark and frightening. When a candle is lighted the room gives up its ghastly secret; it is piled high with blood, offal, and blackened bones. The sisters shut the door and run, but trouble follows them. The little key begins to bleed great drops of blood, streams of blood, that cannot be stanched, so it is hidden away. When Bluebeard returns and asks for his key ring, he knows immediately what has happened and announces that the bones belong to his previous wives, whom he has murdered. When he tells his young wife that she is next, she begs for fifteen minutes to compose herself and make her peace before being beheaded. In that time she calls out repeatedly to her sisters, asking whether their brothers have arrived yet. Just in the nick of time the brothers come and slay Bluebeard.*

Clarissa Pinkola Estés likens Bluebeard to an inner voice that claims we are never enough, a voice that constantly diminishes our creativity and power. This voice comes from two sources. First, the societal stereotypes of women as the weaker sex, the Traditional Homemaker, are present in every woman, no matter how "liberated" she may be. Second, the majority of women in their thirties are still struggling with the adolescent dilemma of reclaiming their own voice by being able to do what they need to do without feeling as if they are being selfish toward others. Bluebeard is the sum total of the inner voices and beliefs that keep a young woman from coming into her own.

Naturally this inner Bluebeard often attracts its match from the outer world and constructs a drama that plays out the intense intrapsychic energies. The young wife in the story represents the creative energy within a woman's soul which, in its naïveté, tries to borrow power and prestige from a man. A woman whose early life structure is that of the Homemaker enters into a bargain to do just that. She supports the man behind the scenes and derives her own prestige for caring for his home and children, entertaining business guests or serving beer to his buddies, helping him advance in the world. The Career Woman derives prestige in typically male-dominated enterprises by taking on the psychological characteristics of men, masculinizing her-

---

*From *Women Who Run with the Wolves: Myths and Stories of the Wild Woman Archetype*, by Clarissa Pinkola Estés, Ph.D. New York: Ballantine Books, © 1992, 1995, pp. 40–44, with the kind permission of Dr. Estés and her publishers.

self to get ahead. The unwritten rules for a woman in a man's world is to be tough, independent, and show little or no emotion. The process of handing over our power to the inner masculine archetype of Bluebeard, the archetype that wishes to keep us in submissive positions, dampens the intuitive knowledge that this is a lethal choice. The more injured we are in childhood, and the more in need of external verification, the more unconscious we are of our own inner life and the more in danger of Bluebeard's power.

Bluebeard forbids the use of one little key, the key to consciousness, to self-awareness, and thus to freedom. For the young woman who may have been abused in childhood, for example, opening this door is indeed like coming into a room full of blood and bones. And for each of us who has laid aside hopes and dreams, settling for being less than we are, carnage also lies behind the door. The key represents a question that a woman must ask in order to learn from the past, redeem it, and use it as compost for growth and empowerment. Estés writes of four basic questions that a woman like Liza, finding herself in a Bluebeard situation, must ask: "What stands behind? What is not as it appears? What do I know deep in my ovaries that I wish I did not know? What of me has been killed, or lays dying?"

Ultimately, once the door to the inner darkness was opened, Bluebeard's young wife rapidly lost her naïveté and used her wiles to stall her murderous husband until help came. The brothers, of course, represent the young woman's own positive inner masculine powers that enable her to act autonomously in the world with integrity and happiness, without compromising her feminine values of relationality, cooperation, and interdependence.

Overcoming Bluebeard is the gift of the age thirty transition. Julia's Bluebeard became obvious when the stress of caring for a second child disturbed the balance of her life. Before Benjamin was born she had conformed to the Homemaker archetype. While she enjoyed and valued her job as a social worker, a career in a "nurture field" that is woman dominated, her primary goals were caring for her family and supporting her physician husband in his work. When a fussy baby left her feeling exhausted and over the edge, she had to reconsider what was most important to her. Should she take a few years off and stay home with the children? Would she miss adult companionship and the challenge of her job if she did? Would taking time off interfere with her plans to become a professor of social work and perhaps eventually the chairperson of her department?

Julia and Roger had to clarify their mutual wants and needs, and renegotiate their marriage arrangement to put Julia on a track that was in line with her newly emergent life structure. Whereas previously home had been the central concern of her life, she decided that career and home were actually coequal concerns and that Roger would have to step up his involvement with the children in order for her to remain happy and creative. Fortunately, Roger was willing and able to arrange his life as a family practice physician around a schedule that left some time to help with child care. Both Julia and Roger arranged to work four-day weeks so that the children would only need to be with a child-care provider for three days. This arrangement helped the irritable Benjamin to calm down, giving him more of a sense of continuity. It also served as a symbol of a new parity in care of the family and importance of career.

The central question that drove Liza's age thirty transition centered on whether working in a male-dominated occupation was worth the toll it took on her creativity and health. She wanted a child and was beginning to realize that the intense work stress might be contributing to her inability to conceive. The question became one of what kind of work would be fulfilling, make use of her prior training and experience, and be less stressful. She decided to leave the track of overall hospital administration, where her eventual goal would have been to become a vice president or CEO. If she really wanted to effect change in hospitals, she reasoned, why not work in the employee assistance program, trying to introduce new health benefits and innovative programs for stress management? If hospital workers felt better that should translate to better care for the patients.

Between the years 1960 and 1992, women's participation in the U.S. labor force rose from 38 to 45 percent. Sixty-eight percent of women are employed in the service and trade industries, a fact that is often attributed to discrimination that keeps women out of higher-echelon professions. While there is no question that such discrimination exists, and must be remediated, it is also important to consider the possibility that some women prefer service sector jobs for a variety of practical, psychological, and spiritual reasons. A friend of mine who was a very successful lawyer, for instance, had an emotional "crash" in her late thirties characterized by the sudden breakthrough of traumatic memories. The process of healing brought up questions concerning the meaning of life, deep spiritual questions. She decided to retrain as a therapist, a "service" position lower on the social power hierarchy than a lawyer, but one in accord with her emerging spirituality.

The gift of the age thirty transition is a values clarification, the first of several that occur throughout the feminine life cycle. What is important? What is the measure of success? What is our legacy to ourselves, our children, and the world?

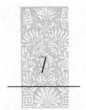

AGES 35–42: HEALING AND BALANCE

SPINNING STRAW INTO GOLD

Julia, at thirty-eight, is a professional career woman. She has just been promoted to full professor at the college of social work where she teaches, and continues her clinical work as a hospital social worker who counsels women on birth control and reproductive problems. Her children, Amanda and Benjamin, are eleven and seven, and she has been married to Roger for thirteen years. As for most working mothers, time is a perpetual issue for Julia. On her good days life seems full, meaningful, and rich. On her bad days she feels like a rat running endlessly around a wheel that never comes to a stop long enough for her to regroup and catch her breath.

The biggest emotional problem for Julia is her marriage. Once primary, it has become a more distant priority, and she misses the excitement and emotional closeness of the early days when she and Roger were building a new life together. Their weekend activities are child centered; a continuous round of chauffeuring the kids to sports, Cub

Scouts, friends' houses, and a variety of cultural activities that they have agreed are important. Their sex life is intermittent at best, and although Julia has kept herself attractive and in good shape, she wonders whether Roger still finds her desirable. With all the emphasis on children and career, there is little time for romance. Worse still, Julia has begun to wonder if Roger might be having an affair with his office manager, Stacey, a witty, outgoing blond woman in her midtwenties. He seems so emotionally distant. Afraid to confront him directly with her fears, Julia has begun to make innuendoes about Stacey, commenting on how beautiful she is and how much time Roger seems to spend on call at nights lately. She's irritable, picking on Roger for little things like forgetting to pick up the dry cleaning or put away the dishes from his bedtime snack. He, in turn, has begun sniping at Julia and complaining that she's always trying to control him and get her own way. As a result, the two are growing progressively more distant.

THE CULMINATING LIFE STRUCTURE
OF YOUNG ADULTHOOD

By their early forties, women have completed the three seven-year cycles that comprise the two decades of young adulthood, a time during which they have tested what Daniel Levinson calls their entry life structure, readjusted it on the basis of the age thirty transition, and then developed a culminating life structure for the first third of their adult lives. Julia's culminating life structure is built on the coequality of family and career, and she continues to juggle many responsibilities, keenly aware that the archetype of the Superwoman is a difficult life structure to maintain. Furthermore, the quality of her marriage is deteriorating, calling her attention not only to rebalancing priorities but also to the necessity for some emotional healing work. The fact that she can't confront Roger directly with her fear that he is having an affair, but instead drops sarcastic hints, is an old pattern. Whenever relationships are going poorly in her life, Julia tends to feel rejected and blame the other person. Instead, she needs to learn that periods of conflict in relationships are to be expected. They can be great opportunities for growth and self-awareness, but only if both people are willing to communicate their feelings and thoughts openly and with respect. Avoiding difficult conversations, an emotional style she learned from her mother, Sylvia, just allows negative feelings to build up, creating unnecessary damage and undermining the self-esteem of both parties.

In this chapter we will focus on the opportunity that women like Julia have to resolve two major problems that may keep them from enjoying the life structures they have so carefully put into place: making new priorities and completing prior developmental phases that we may not yet have fully mastered. This latter opportunity involves work on emotional healing. The need for healing often becomes evident when recurring problems in relationships signal that something within us needs to be put right. I often call this work of converting old wounds to wisdom, spinning straw into gold. It is a transformation of something old and worthless into something precious and enduring. If we balance priorities and heal old emotional scars by the end of early adulthood, we will be in the best possible position to go through the metamorphosis of midlife and continue on the trajectory of authenticity, relationality, power, and service that are key to the last half of the feminine life cycle.

DIVORCE, MODERN FAMILY PATTERNS, AND THE CULMINATING LIFE STRUCTURE OF YOUNG ADULTHOOD

While Julia and Roger are experiencing a nadir in their relationship, neither one is thinking about divorce, making them a minority among couples marrying today. The divorce rate has climbed from about 10 percent for couples married in 1920, to 50 percent for those married in 1970, to a projected 67 percent of those married in 1990. In trying to answer the question "Why do people divorce?" anthropologist Helen Fisher focuses not only on quarrels, insensitivity, and disrespect, but on two key sociobiological factors: adultery and infertility. In a study of 160 cultures worldwide, the wife's adultery or inability to bear children headed the list of reasons for divorce, validating Darwin's hypothesis that people marry primarily as a way of procreating and protecting their offspring. Other data also reinforce Darwin's point of view. For example, a United Nations study of hundreds of millions of people from 45 societies found that "39 percent of all divorces occurred among couples with no dependent children, 26 percent among those with one dependent child, 19 percent among couples with two 'issue,' 7 percent among those with three children, 3 percent among couples with four young, and couples with five or more dependent children rarely split. Hence it appears that the more children a couple bear, the less likely they are to divorce."

Anthropologist Helen Fisher reasons that the biological urge to reproduce is behind these data since couples without children can find new mates and bear young, while those with many children stand a better chance of caring for them economically by staying together. Many of the divorced women in Levinson's sample, in contrast to the United Nations data, did have children to care for, indicating that in modern America, sociobiological concerns about children are often overridden by a couple's psychological or physical (in cases of abuse) need to separate. One obvious reason that Americans buck the sociobiological trend is that the relative wealth of Americans, even of those who are poor, is much greater than in many other countries. Even though it can be extremely difficult for single mothers with children to survive financially, they still have substantially more resources than mothers in Third World countries. Additionally, the rise of the archetypal Antitraditional Figure in modern women's lives makes it less likely that a woman will subjugate her physical or mental health to maintain a traditional (nondivorced) family structure.

The peak time of divorce for women is while they are in their late twenties and early thirties after an average of four years of marriage. So while divorce rates are highest during the age thirty transition, they continue at a high level throughout the thirties. In Levinson's study, for example, over half the women (eight out of fifteen) in his homemaker sample experienced serious marital problems in their thirties. Two women had already divorced in their twenties. Three more got legally divorced in their thirties and another five "gave up on" their husbands and continued to live in poor, distanced relationships. Of these, three more got legal divorces during the next several years. In the career woman sample, twelve of thirty women were in their first marriage by the end of the culminating life structure period in their early forties. Five were in second marriages, and nine were divorced. Four of the thirty had never married.

The number of families headed by single mothers has grown dramatically over the last two decades, keeping pace with the increased divorce rates and demonstrating that children are not always a sufficient reason to keep marriages together. In 1970 10.9 percent of all American households consisted of a single mother and her children. By 1991 that number had risen to 17.4 percent. Economically, such families are at a decided disadvantage since their average income is only about two fifths that of married couples in which both husband and wife work and slightly less than half that of married couples in which only the husband works. Nonetheless, the interviews that Levinson's group conducted clearly indicated that women in their thirties were happier to take their chances with economic insecurity than they were to continue in hurtful or loveless relationships, particularly those in which the husband was an outright philanderer, drunk, drug abuser, or unable or unwilling to help support the family financially. As women moved into the culminating period of their entry life structure, they were increasingly clear that husbands who didn't contribute to their life plan had to go.

The determination to divorce is never an easy one, but the gradual strengthening of the archetype that Levinson calls the Antitraditional Figure helps women make that choice. By the end of a woman's thirties, the gap between the entry life structures of the homemaker and career woman sample had substantially narrowed. The homemakers were less interested in a life predicated on the continuing care of others, and more interested in finding creative, affirming lives for themselves, as the career women had been from the outset. Many tended to move out of the traditional marriage mode in which the wife cares for the husband and children, into a modified marriage mode where an equal partnership was more to their liking. While divorce was not a necessary part of that shift, it was a reality for a substantial number of women by the time they reached their early forties. But the question that remains after a divorce is whether or not we have learned anything from our experience that will aid us in becoming wiser, more compassionate, more emotionally whole human beings.

HEALING INTO RELATIONSHIP

Helen Luke, an Oxford-educated psychologist, writes in *The Way of Woman*, "If we break vows for any other reason than out of obedience to a more compelling loyalty, then the situation from which we have tried to escape will simply repeat itself in another form. Nonetheless, for thousands of men and women who take the marriage vow in sincerity, the test of daily life through the years makes it plain that the choice they made was conditioned by projections which, as they fade, leave exposed the fact that the two personalities are, or have become, destructive of one another. . . ."

Pick up a morning newspaper in almost any city, and tucked away on the back page you're likely to read a story like this one, published in the *Denver Post*. A twenty-seven-year-old man was badly burned when the woman he was living with poured a bottle of rubbing alcohol over his head and lit him with a match. The reason? He had forgotten to stop at the store for a quart of milk. While the milk was probably the last straw in an unpublished list of grievances, the article was written in a way that summoned up some of my own feelings of frustration about the Herculean, and often unacknowledged, efforts that many women make to manage a house, work, and care for their children. The Denver woman was obviously upset and wished her man would help, but she approached the problem in a terrible way, revealing in Helen Luke's words just how destructive she and her boyfriend had become of each other.

Psychologist Daniel Goleman has made an excellent case for the lack of emotional intelligence in our country, yet unlike the Denver woman, most of us try our best to get along with others. The problem is that the difficulties we encounter in our most intimate relationships don't occur in a vacuum. They often have their roots in a history of past hurts and erroneous beliefs that have literally become part of our nervous systems. If in childhood, for example, we had parents who settled disputes with violence, when we experience rage as adults, our limbic system will tend to discharge it along well-myelinated pathways leading to the frontal lobes. The frontal lobes will determine that violence is a socially acceptable response, and like the Denver woman we will be prone to redress our grievances through aggression.

There's an old saying that you can't fix what you don't know is broken. In the case of the young woman who set her boyfriend on fire, something was obviously broken. But for many of us, the signs are subtler, and like Julia we may be well on into our thirties before we begin to identify subtle patterns of behavior that are compromising the quality of our relationships. Such patterns have been the subject of intensive research, particularly at the University of Washington in Seattle.

For over twenty years the University of Washington has been investigating the psychological and physiological aspects of relationship. Informally dubbed "the love lab," the Family Formation Project is headed by mathematician-turned-psychologist John Gottman. Concerned that most marriage counseling lacked a scientific basis, Gottman and his colleagues set out to define the characteristics of healthy relationships so that therapy could be more effective. Making liberal use of videotaping and physiological monitoring, Gottman has fed mounds of data to computers. Like psychological X-rays, the results are a remarkably effective indicator of the longevity of relationships. With an astounding 94 percent rate of accuracy, Gottman and his colleagues can predict which couples will divorce within four years of testing. Here are some of the most interesting findings compiled from the love lab:

- Healthy relationships, not surprisingly, are based on kindness. Like Roger and Julia in the earlier years of their marriage, the partners are nice to one another *and positive interactions outnumber negative ones at a critical ratio of five to one.* Those headed for divorce, however, have more nasty than nice moments. Since the balance between kindness and criticism is beginning to shift between Julia and Roger, they are at risk for violating this important five-to-one ratio unless they attend to the underlying problems in communication.

- Husbands who do housework are happier, healthier, have better sex lives, and are much more likely to stay married, a fact that many women have intuited but of which husbands may remain unconvinced.

- Women who are married to belittling, contemptuous men are much more likely to fall ill than those w ith supportive spouses. Colds, flu, bladder troubles, yeast infections, and gastrointestinal complaints all mount with lack of respect.

- Disrespectful wives also ruin a marriage. Gottman states that "When a wife's face shows disgust, a near cousin of contempt, four or more times within a fifteen-minute conversation, it is a silent sign that the couple is likely to separate within four years."

Ideally, relationships are the ground for emotional and spiritual growth as well as a place for healing. But we can't heal unless we know we are broken. So when disagreements occur, particularly those in which the body reacts strongly, we have a clue that healing is needed. Couples who are in rapport with each other actually entrain each other's autonomic nervous systems. When one partner gets stressed and anxious, the other is likely to follow. But if one partner begins to relax, the other is also likely to calm down, allowing rational thinking to modulate emotions. The psychobiological feedback loop operates not only within our own bodies, but also between a woman and her significant other, and a woman and her children.

Within every person there is both light and shadow, that which heals and that which, when left unattended, destroys. In the beginning of a relationship we see one another's light, but with time our mutual shadows begin to creep out. For example, when Julia and Roger first married, he seemed to be a mild-mannered man with whom she got along quite well, until gradually he started to accuse her of being critical. Little by little, incident by incident, Julia did start to feel angry and critical. Roger's part of the unconscious dynamic was this. Somewhere in his childhood, he internalized the message that anger was unacceptable, learning to repress it so that it wouldn't cause overt anxiety. When Roger gets angry, the impulse rarely reaches his conscious mind, but somewhere deep in his limbic system a kind of projector begins to run. Instead of experiencing the emotion personally, he literally sees its image outside of himself. Julia appears to him to be an angry, critical person.

Projection of one's shadow is an example of negative empathy. In an unconscious collusion, Julia ends up experiencing Roger's repressed feelings. Family therapist Virginia Satir compared the hidden impulses of the shadow to a pack of hungry dogs scratching at the cellar door. It takes a lot of energy to keep the door shut. It is also incredibly draining to cope with the hurt feelings and tangled emotions that occur when so many of our perceptions and behaviors are unconscious. No wonder that fatigue of "unknown etiology" (medicalese meaning "for no apparent reason") is the number-one health complaint for women.

Julia's body told the story of the deterioration of their marriage through fatigue, headaches, and low back pain. But instead of continuing to blame Roger for all their problems, dooming herself to repeat similar relationships with others, she finally took responsibility for her own behavior and sought therapy. Levinson's research indicates that half of his career woman sample sought therapy sometime in their thirties, a much larger proportion than in the homemaker sample. Although the career women were no more troubled, they were aware that their problems might be easier to solve with some outside help.

In therapy, Julia complained that Roger rarely helped around the house, but she also realized that she gave him little opportunity because her own perfectionism made it impossible to leave the dishes in the sink long enough for him to get around to them. It bothered her that he was a workaholic and yet she enabled him to continue by putting aside her own desire or need to work a little harder, or see friends, instead staying home with the kids while Roger put in extra time at the office. Unresolved problems in the adolescent stage of the life cycle had left Julia with boundary issues. The questions "Where do I begin and others end?" and "How can I get my own needs met without being selfish?" had not yet been answered. Therapy helped her work through this issue and come to the realization that better communication was a cornerstone of change. She couldn't expect Roger to be a mind reader. She had to make her needs and feelings known.

Julia finally confronted Roger about her fears that he was having an affair with his office manager. She was surprised when he burst out laughing. He had similar suspicions about Julia, whose warm relationship with the dean of the college had often made him jealous. In talking about their feelings, both were reassured and the escalating fears of rejection diminished on both parts. Self-awareness is a gift of growth potentially present in all conflicts. But it is up to each one of us, like Julia, to accept that gift and use it as the basis for moving into authentic, mutually growth-enhancing relationships with self and others.

Psychiatrist Jean Baker Miller, founder of Wellesley College's Stone Center for Women's Studies, has commented that women try to bring forth the best in themselves and others in all relationships. In her classic text *Toward a New Psychology of Women*, she writes that even within the context of abusive or violent relationships women continue to develop valuable psychological characteristics because they "struggle to create growth-fostering interactions within the family and in other settings." I believe that this struggle, and the fact that we continue to grow in relationality even in suboptimal relationships, accounts for the fact that many women choose to stay in difficult marriages for prolonged periods of time.

But as women mature and become more emotionally astute, inauthentic relationships become harder to abide. A woman's core essence, after all, is defined by relationality, specifically by the concept of self-in-relation, which means that we feel most at home in our skin when relationships are characterized by each partner bringing forth something new in the other. By the end of our young adulthood we are less willing to tolerate one-way relationships that are not mutually growth enhancing because we clearly perceive that they are out of accord with our essential nature. When we cannot resolve our differences and come into a new, more honest, and respectful relationship as Julia and Roger did, we are faced with the need to terminate the relationship, which, precisely because of our investment in relationality, is often a difficult choice for a woman to make, particularly if she still has any of her own emotional healing work to complete.

WOMEN AND ABUSE

While as in Julia's case healing is often a matter of going back and completing an earlier developmental stage, many women have a more intense type of healing to accomplish. In 1980 sociologist Diana Russell interviewed more than nine hundred women, chosen at random, about their experiences of sexual assault and domestic violence. The results were horrifying. One woman in four had been raped, and one woman in three had been sexually abused in childhood. Furthermore, it is likely that abuse is underreported, both because some women don't want to admit to it, and also because memories of abuse are often repressed until a woman is in her late thirties or early forties. A study at Boston City Hospital in the early 1970s identified "rape trauma syndrome," a constellation of symptoms consisting of physical complaints, anxiety, depression, flashbacks, phobic fears, and sleep disturbances including nightmares that appear not only in women who have been raped as adults, but in many women who were abused as children.

While healing from abuse is not normally considered a developmental stage in the life cycle of women, perhaps it should be. Not only is the prevalence of physical and sexual abuse striking, but emotional abuse and poor parenting are practically endemic in our culture. Another reason for considering emotional healing as a predictable part of the closing cycle of young adulthood rests on clinical experience. Many therapists have noted that women who were abused in childhood, and who have coped reasonably well throughout their twenties and early thirties, often suddenly "crash" in their late thirties and early forties and begin a cycle of healing. Furthermore, 25 percent of us, no matter how idyllic our childhood or adult life, can expect to have our lives suddenly and dramatically changed by rape. Whether the victim is ourself, our mother, our daughter, or a friend, it is a rare woman who goes through the life cycle untouched by this particular tragedy.

"Robbie," for example, was a client referred to me when I directed the Mind/Body Clinic at Boston's Beth Israel Hospital. She was hysterical the first time we met, tears flowing down her wan cheeks. At thirty-four she looked fifty, and a tired, listless fifty at that. She had been referred to me for stress reduction by a therapist at the hospital's rape crisis intervention center. While her reaction was not at all unusual for a woman who had recently been raped, Robbie's trauma had occurred nearly two years earlier. But even now she had trouble falling asleep, and when she did was often awakened by nightmares that seemed like instant replays of the assault. Robbie also described episodes in which she would just "numb out," staring at the wall for hours. She startled easily, her concentration was disturbed, she was having trouble meeting deadlines at the advertising agency where she worked, and she was bothered by chronic stomach pains. Although Robbie's symptoms were severe, I have treated hundreds of women with milder variants of the same symptoms, often called post-traumatic stress disorder or PTSD.

THE PHYSIOLOGY OF TRAUMATIC MEMORIES

For more than a hundred years scientists have noted that the psychological effects of trauma are often somaticized, or experienced in the body. Many women who sought help at the Mind/Body Clinic for chronic pain syndromes such as fibrositis (an autoimmune condition in which the body attacks components of its connective tissue creating painful inflammation) had childhood histories of physical or sexual abuse. In the late 1800s the psychiatrist Pierre Janet hypothesized that the intense emotions evoked by painful situations cause memories of the trauma to be repressed. They are experienced instead as sensations of fear, physical manifestations (these include rare and striking symptoms such as hysterical blindness and paralysis as well as common stress-related disorders like irritable bowel syndrome, stomach aches, headaches, high blood pressure, irregular heartbeats, and back pain) or visual images such as nightmares and flashbacks.

Repression can occur because there are two types of memory. The usual kind is called semantic or declarative memory, which is stored in the words through which we recall events. This storytelling mode of memory hinges on the ability to verbalize our experience, encode the memory traces in a part of the brain called the hippocampus, and then consciously fit the memory into the scheme of our existing experiences. Since semantic memory doesn't occur until we are old enough to speak, we can't generally recall much before the age of three or four. We do, however, have memories of that time encoded in a different system that stores images, or icons, of our experience. This early childhood memory system relies on the amygdala, which is also the storage site for all emotionally charged or traumatic memories. The icons, or visual representations, do not fade over time as semantic memory often does. And while semantic memory falters under stress, iconic memories surface: whereas semantic memories are linear and rational, iconic memories are timeless. They are as strong today as they were when they were first engraved by the neurotransmitters within the amygdala. In sleep the higher cortical mechanisms that control the breakthrough of iconic memory weaken, resulting in nightmares and flashbacks of the repressed trauma. Our conscious censors also weaken as we age, which may explain the breakthrough of traumatic memories that commonly occurs in the late thirties and forties.

The existence of iconic memory leaves us open to being retraumatized whenever a current situation reminds us of the past, or whenever we experience stress of any kind. Bessel Van der Kolk, a Harvard psychiatrist who is an expert on abuse and trauma, writes, "Under ordinary conditions traumatized people, including rape victims, battered women and abused children have a fairly good psychosocial adjustment. However, they do not respond to stress in the way that other people do. Under pressure they may feel or act as if they were being traumatized all over again. Thus high states of arousal seem selectively to promote retrieval of traumatic memories."

The retrieval of the memory, or the physiological response to it, escalates the stress further. This positive feedback loop further strengthens the original memory trace, explaining why some people who have coped reasonably well in adult life suddenly "crash" from a stressful situation that would seem insufficient to produce such a strong response. This loop has been compared to a "black hole" in the emotional circuitry that attracts every related event to itself and destroys the quality of life.

The black hole effect can lead to the sudden appearance of phobic fear and terrible distress in a person who may have seemed well adjusted. An apparently normal woman, for example, might suddenly "freak out" and become hysterically paralyzed when she cannot calm down a screaming toddler who is having a tantrum. As the child's emotional stress escalates, so does the mother's until her nervous system is in a high state of excitation. The shrieks of the child, coupled with her own high nervous system arousal, plug in to memory circuits laid down when she was abused as a child. A relationship in which angry fights begin to flare up may similarly lead to the seemingly unrelated appearance of PTSD.

The physiology of trauma also provides insights into why people often stay in abusive situations. It is easy for an outsider to criticize a battered woman who continues to live with her abuser. But research on both mice and humans indicates that when the nervous system is hyperaroused—as it is in any situation where we must constantly be vigilant for danger—we will seek that which is most familiar regardless of the outcome. For example, a mouse who is locked in a box, given electric shocks, and then released will return to the box when it is stressed. Interestingly, stroking the mouse actually helps it overcome its tendency to seek safety in danger, and to learn new responses.

What about the woman who keeps on falling for abusive men? While her semantic memory serves her well, and she recalls how miserable she was with the last no-good dirty dog, her iconic memory leads her to recreate the familiar pain over and over again. The most important question here is, how can we extinguish those pesky iconic memory traces? One way is repeatedly to verbalize our problems, talking them through with friends, a therapist, or in a journal. This helps transfer iconic memories into semantic ones over which we have much greater control. Some trauma victims naturally do this, telling and retelling their stories. When my father, ill with cancer, ended his life by jumping from a thirty-seventh-story window, my mother was emotionally devastated. She told and retold her story to anyone who would listen. Some of the family became concerned that the constant repetition would do her more harm than good. But speaking and being listened to heals. It actually changes our neural circuitry, as does touch.

To speak, to be heard, and to be held are basic to healing, as is the creation of meaning. Psychiatrist Viktor Frankl, writing of the unspeakable horrors of the Nazi concentration camps in which he was imprisoned for several years, cited the primary importance of meaning to survival. Those prisoners who could find no meaning for their suffering were much more likely to fall ill and die than were those who could construct some positive framework for their suffering.

The old adage "That which doesn't kill me makes me stronger" is a wonderful starting point for meaning. Every human being experiences some trauma in the course of her life, and in the healing can grow in wisdom and compassion. A young friend with severe manic depressive illness helped herself greatly with the strong belief that the illness was a divine gift that had opened her heart to other people whom she would someday be able to help as a therapist. Another friend of mine who is a therapist was a severely abused child. She actually recalls an angelic visitation after one particularly hideous beating in which she was told that she would heal and grow up to help others.

CAREER AND MEANING

Many women who have healed old traumas during this young adult passage do, in fact, seek new careers in which the gifts of compassion and wisdom that they have claimed can be used to help other people. When I lecture on mind/body medicine, healing, and spirituality around the country—both to professionals and to the general public— approximately 80 percent of the attendees are women, as are many of the presenters. The peak age range for attendees is midthirties through midfifties; women who are either in the process of healing or women who have done a great deal of healing and now feel compelled to share their psychological and spiritual growth with others.

There is a profound and increasingly popular psychospiritual heal- ing movement in our country, and women in the culminating stages of young adulthood, and those in midlife, are at its core. It is not surpris- ing that the primary tenets of physical, emotional, and spiritual healing concern relationality, specifically a person's relationship to herself, to other people, and to the cosmos. When I am giving a lecture or work- shop on healing and spirituality, I often ask for a show of hands from those who have had some life experience of physical or psychological wounding, and have subsequently decided to dedicate their lives to helping others. The great majority of women in the group wave their hands enthusiastically. Carl Jung wrote of the archetype called the Wounded Healer, making the point that we develop empathy in the process of healing that helps us to become more intuitive, compassion- ate therapists. Since women are already empathetic and intuitive, the healing process results in a further development of gifts that are al- ready part of our psychological and neurological makeup.

As we continue to heal and grow in life experience, the questions that come into focus are the value-related ones that a woman reviews many times in the course of her life, such as "What is the purpose of human life?" "What is the meaning of success?" "What is the measure of a life well lived?" These are all questions that relate back to the em- phasis on relationality and interdependence that define the psycho- spiritual nature of women. Both as a therapist and workshop leader, I have heard a common story from a large number of women in their midthirties and forties. The intuitive spirituality of interconnectedness has always been present, but even after the adolescent awakening to self-in-relation, there is another cycle of falling asleep to it in young adulthood when issues like establishing an independent life, settling on a career, beginning relationships, and bearing children take practical precedence. Several of the women in Levinson's sample described this experience as "being in a fog." As a woman in one of my workshops said, the twenties and most of the thirties are the "full-steam-ahead, damn-the-torpedos years," and there's hardly time to catch a breath. Then, as we mature and especially when we experience traumas, disappointments, failures, the death of parents and other losses, the spiritual questions of meaning come into bold relief. The cyclic periods of questioning that women go through lead to periodic reassessment of priorities, another important feature of the thirties and early forties.

OUTER BALANCE: REVIEWING PRIORITIES

Following the therapy that Julia and Roger underwent, they both decided to make their relationship as important a priority as it was in the early days of their marriage. They made a date to go out by themselves, or with friends, at least once a week. They also made plans to take a long weekend together, without the children, at least four times a year. Perhaps most important, they broke the habit of getting into bed and burying their noses in separate books. Instead, they spent the last half hour of each day listening to one another, and sometimes giving the more tired one a short massage. The latter activity, they soon discovered, often led to cuddling, kissing, and sometimes to intercourse. Both of them realized how starved they had been for touch, and how easy it was to confuse the need for touch with the need for sex. Both were important, but previously, when most of their touch needs had to be satisfied with sex, they got neither. Having intercourse had often seemed like a burden at the end of a long day, so it rarely happened. It was a surprise and a delight to discover that sex often unfolded organically from touching and hugging. When it was no longer a "should," it became a much more regular source of intimacy and pleasure.

Julia's concern with time, specifically the perception that there was never enough of it, was also partially driven by "shoulds." By constantly telling herself that she should have more time for this or that, that her life was out of balance, she made negatives out of positives. Why complain that the work she loved was using up all her time? Didn't she choose that work, devoting years to training for it? Why complain about the complexity of caring for the children? Hadn't she wanted children to care for since she was a little girl? She's done what she could to balance her priorities, making more time for her marriage, and she still wishes that there was more time for seeing friends and slipping away by herself, but there isn't. No person's life is perfect, at least for long, and it is the rare individual who has everything she wants.

Many women complain bitterly about being too busy, about having too little time. But being busy is a given for working people, especially working mothers who, research indicates, still do much more housework and child care than their working husbands. Solving the problem has two prongs: rebalancing priorities when necessary, and changing our attitude about being busy. In recent years busy women have too often been labeled as unbalanced workaholics. Many books tout the benefits of taking more time for ourselves, and suggest that if we don't, we're psychologically or spiritually in the wrong. While it is crucial for women to take some time each day for themselves to recharge, it is often impossible to take very much. But perhaps we don't need very much. I know that even a few minutes of prayer or meditation rejuvenates me as does caring for my houseplants, walking through the garden, calling a friend, taking a walk, doing a little yoga, or reading a book. The problem is that many books suggest that I should be able to do all of those things most every day, scolding me if I don't. If I believed them I'd feel very guilty for ignoring myself, a guilt which many women now experience.

In thinking about why women are making one another feel guilty about being busy, it is interesting to reflect upon our mothers' generation. My mother, for example, was molded in the form of Betty Friedan's "feminine mystique." Mom got her prestige by borrowing it from a man, and to her the most important things for a successful woman were a rich mate, prestige items like expensive clothing, a nice house and car, lots of leisure time, running a tip-top house with beautiful, well-behaved children, and having time for volunteer work in the community. In my mother's day, what Daniel Levinson called the archetypal Traditional Homemaker Figure was in its heyday.

In *The Seasons of a Woman's Life*, Levinson quotes a lecture that English novelist Virginia Woolf delivered to a group of professional women in 1931, when she was forty-nine years old. Her topic was the "inner phantoms" that sparred in her psyche and how they affected her creative life. Her name for the Traditional Homemaker Figure was the Angel of the House. Her Angel was the perfect example of the feminine mystique—demure, self-sacrificing, caring more for the needs of others than her own, and deriving power by borrowing it from a man. The Angel of the House was always whispering instructions to Woolf on how to write, instructions that would have caused the famous novelist to lose her voice in service of remaining socially acceptable. Woolf had to face this part of herself head-on. She spoke of doing her best to kill the Angel, to strangle it, in self-defense. For otherwise it would choke off her creative life and deprive her of having a mind of her own.

Woolf hoped that the next generation of women would be free from the constraining voice of the Angel of the House, able to speak their minds and follow their dreams into every kind of human endeavor. But we are not free from the Angel and her constant struggles with our creative selves, the Antitraditional Figure. The inner and outer voices that criticize the busy woman for being out of balance, for having too little time for herself or her friends and family, are a chorus of Angels of the House, Traditional Homemaker Figures. The perfect woman of Virginia Woolf's generation, and my mother's after hers, was supposed to have plenty of time for leisure, family, and friendship pursuits. The Angel's admonitions haven't changed over the years, only her clothing has. Now she wears the vestments of a kind of generic spirituality, and utters instructions on how to live a perfectly balanced life as a kind of Angelic Traditional Priestess. Her spiritual garb makes her gibes particularly sharp, since she pretends to hold the true keys to our happiness.

I am often the target of projection for women's Traditional Homemaker Figures. Many friends and even women that I've just met at workshops cluck their tongues at me and express their sadness that my life is so busy and out of balance. I should have more time for myself, for friends, for family. The fact is that my new marriage is a priority to which I devote plenty of time, and that I have a very close network of women friends to whom I also devote a lot of time. Because I travel about two hundred days a year, much of that time is on the phone from airports and hotel rooms, but we continue to have close, supportive relationships. An additional benefit of travel is that I get to visit my children, who live across the country, quite frequently, as well as friends and relatives in different locations. Time on airplanes is not a problem; it is a joy. There is uninterrupted time to read, meditate, nap, write, and generally unwind.

There are, of course, compromises. I love to hike and spend time in nature, which is why I live in a mountain wilderness area. Because of my traveling, I spend less time there than I might otherwise. But overall I have few complaints. My work is incredibly rich and satisfying, I feel as though I'm being of service, the pay is good, and I chose it. There are certainly days when I wish I could be on vacation, when I feel overwhelmed. Everyone has those days. But overall I feel sincerely grateful for the opportunity to live such an interesting, varied life. Having confronted my Traditional Homemaker Figure and seen through her attempts to make me feel guilty, I am free to enjoy the life I worked so hard to create.

Life is difficult and complex both for today's homemaker, who often works outside the home, and for today's career woman, who often maintains a family. Let's support one another in the knowledge that, as both the Wellesley College Lifeprints Study and Levinson's study have shown, complex lives are not unhappy lives. The highest level of life satisfaction found in the Lifeprints Study was among the busiest women in the sample, working mothers. Busy is an opportunity, not a dirty word. One of the main pleasures of busy working women, not surprisingly, is the relatively large number of relationships that can develop in the work setting, as opposed to the relatively isolated existence of a woman who stays home. We are happiest when the opportunities for experiencing self-in-relation are greatest. There may be stress in multiple roles, but there is also the satisfaction of interacting in multiple ways with a myriad of people who bring out parts of ourselves of which we may have been previously unaware.

INNER BALANCE

The idea that our lives should be balanced is a good one, but there is a big difference between outer balance and inner balance. Outer balance fluctuates with the needs of the day and the year, and how best to maintain the life structures we have worked so hard to put in place. But within each day, no matter its mix of tasks and pleasures, we can maintain an inner balance. When we are capable of living in the moment free from the tyranny of "shoulds," free from the nagging sensation that this moment isn't right, we will have peaceful hearts.

My colleague, Dr. Jon Kabat-Zinn, director of the Center for Mindfulness and Medicine at the University of Massachusetts Medical School, has written extensively on mindfulness, or the nonjudgmental awareness of the present moment. Mindfulness is a natural pleasure, a natural state of creativity and union with a larger whole. But most of us are rarely mindful. Instead, we tend to be mindless. The lights are on, but nobody's home. For example, what's the use of making love if your mind is on a presentation due at work or a problem you are having with a child? Where's the pleasure in eating a piece of chocolate cake if you're so busy watching television that you don't notice the cake's fragrance, texture, and taste?

As we age, there is a tendency to ask questions about meaning, about happiness. The hope is that by the end of her thirties a woman has clarified her values, adjusted her outer life to be in accord with them, and done whatever emotional healing was necessary to live a happy, productive life. But we may still find that happiness eludes us, that we are habitually elsewhere rather than in the present moment. Particularly when we're so busy it's easy to miss out on appreciating life's many small pleasures—the taste of food, the feeling of the breeze, the colors of a sunset. There are many ways to become more mindful, to reach a more comfortable inner balance. By taking time to pray or meditate, to breathe and mellow out (there is a section on prayer and meditation for you in the Appendix), we can become more attuned to the moment. In doing so, time seems to expand, and we can approach our tasks with a more peaceful heart, open mind, and relaxed attitude.

Prayer and meditation practices have also been proven to reduce stress and enhance health. Harvard cardiologist Herbert Benson, whose

1975 best-seller, *The Relaxation Response,* is a classic, proved that as little as ten to twenty minutes of meditation three or more days per week could reduce anxiety and depression, enhance joy and vitality, and reduce stress-related physical illnesses. When I directed the mind/body programs in Benson's Division of Behavioral Medicine at Boston's New England Deaconess Hospital, I was able to document the positive effects of meditation not only on common stress-related disorders like headache and high blood pressure, but on a wide variety of other medical conditions ranging from insulin-dependent diabetes to asthma to epileptic seizures. The fact is that almost any illness, no matter its cause, can be worsened by stress and improved by methods that restore us to inner balance.

For most women it is helpful to have some ritual, or practice, of coming into the present moment each day. For me, it is prayer. Each morning, when I pray, I enter that timeless moment when there are no boundaries between me and the universe, between past and future. Even when I am very busy, and have just a few minutes to spend in prayer, it helps me to remain mindful throughout the day, so that I can conduct my affairs in balance and in beauty, with guidance from the greater spirit of wisdom and intuition.

When I am in balance, what the Navajos call walking in beauty, I naturally think of the results of my actions. If I don't recycle my bottles, I will harm the earth. To walk in beauty I use what I have, trying not to waste anything. When I am in balance, I don't have to think about doing healthful things for my body, I naturally want to exercise and eat things that make me feel energetic and clear. When I am in balance I am most creative, in harmony with my work. Everything gets done more elegantly, simply, and efficiently because a greater wisdom inspires my thoughts and actions. When I am in balance, I see the best in every situation and feel grateful. My heart is at peace. When I am in balance I see the best in others, and the magic of self-in-relation becomes a reality as each of us comes more fully into being.

THE GIFTS OF THE CULMINATING YEARS OF YOUNG ADULTHOOD

The gift of this final cycle of young adulthood is archetypally portrayed in the fairy tale in which the young heroine must learn to spin straw into gold or else lose her life. No experiences, even difficult ones, are worthless. They can all be spun into gold, giving us gifts of understanding and compassion that were unexpected. A woman who was abused as a child, for example, may find that in the process of grieving the loss of a normal childhood, learning to express her anger, and finally forgiving her parents, she has learned a great deal about human nature that helps her in all her relationships. People are likely to confide in her because her very presence is healing. She exudes a sense of peace and openheartedness and is not prone to judge others. Such a woman has transformed her wounds into wisdom and brought forth the archetype that Jung called the Wounded Healer.

Neuronal pathways that once supported iconic memories of fear can be replaced by semantic pathways that support new memories of healing, connectedness, and positive meaning. This shift from fear to love helps us to build on the core essence of our womanhood, the development of self-in-relation that describes our natural spirituality. The wisdom gained from healing, together with the ability to balance many different life tasks, provides a stable bio-psycho-spiritual feedback loop to support the emergence of the prodigious wisdom that is about to flower as we enter the next cycle of life. The bonus of learning to ignore the guilt-engendering voice of the Traditional Homemaker Figure allows us to be grateful for lives that are full and busy. And the gift of mindfulness helps us to appreciate those busy lives on a moment-by-moment basis that opens us to the intuitive, creative wisdom that has always been within us.

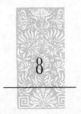

8

AGES 42–49: THE MIDLIFE METAMORPHOSIS

AUTHENTICITY, POWER, AND THE EMERGENCE OF THE GUARDIAN

W hen I was running the Mind/Body Clinic, a forty-five-year-old woman that we'll call Shirley attended one of the cancer groups that I facilitated. She'd had a bilateral mastectomy, but the tumor had already spread to her lymph nodes. Her life was clearly in danger. Midway through the eight-week program she announced to everyone's surprise that she was getting a divorce. At first the group was shocked, and several women jumped to the conclusion that her husband must be leaving her because she had lost both breasts and was no longer desirable to him sexually. Emotion ran high as both the women and the men in the group explored how the changes in their bodies had affected their view of themselves, their relationships with their spouses, or their hopes for future romance. After a while, Shirley broke into the conversation to set matters straight. Her husband had not asked for a divorce, and in fact didn't want one. The decision had been her own because the cancer had given her the opportunity to take a courageous and penetrating look at her life.

It is often crises, particularly those that are life or lifestyle challenging, that bring up the big questions we may have been too busy or preoccupied to think about before. Who are we? What is the meaning and purpose of life? What is happiness? Shirley, the mother of two teenagers, had been contemplating just these questions, not only because she was involved in a life crisis, but also because these questions are a natural part of the reevaluation of our lives that occurs during what psychologist Daniel Levinson calls the midlife transition.

Shirley decided that the most important things in life were love, peace of mind, and service to others, a triad that I believe characterizes the wisdom of the middle-aged woman, and which I call the midlife values triad. Shirley's husband, while not abusive in the common sense of the word, was distant, unsupportive, and openly contemptuous of her desire to go back to school and find a career in the helping professions. Before the cancer she had made excuses for him—after all, he was just an old-fashioned kind of guy, he wanted her to have an easy life at home, the stress in their marriage was her fault for wanting a career. But suddenly, when faced with the possibility of an early death, she realized that the marriage was out of tune with her most cherished values and hopes. Her husband was not about to change, and clearly could not love and support her if she went back to school. It was up to Shirley to decide what was most important, and either adjust to her current circumstances or make the drastic changes that would allow her to live in accord with her most deeply cherished values.

Authenticity arises from a process of self-examination such as the one Shirley underwent that culminates in two outcomes: arriving at a clear set of inner values and then changing one's outer life circumstances to be consonant with them. When our external world reflects and extends our internal values, we reach a state of integrity, or wholeness. In contrast, when inner and outer worlds are not coherent, stress and tension result. Although Shirley understood that leaving her marriage and going back to school would also be stressful, she was right in recognizing that the temporary stress of rising to a challenge that brings us into a larger sense of purpose is far easier than living with the chronic stress of being out of tune with our core beliefs.

Did leaving the marriage and moving into authenticity help Shirley's body fight the cancer? I don't know the answer, but my training in mind/body medicine suggests that it might have. When we feel cut off from ourselves, isolated from other people, nature, or a sense of a greater power, the immune system functions at suboptimal levels. The number and activity of natural killer cells, a kind of lymphocyte that destroys both cancer and virus-infected cells, declines. We look and feel older than we are, drained of vitality and enthusiasm. In the fascinating book *Remarkable Recovery*, writers Caryle Hirshberg and Mark Barasch discuss the commonalities of people who have had spontaneous healings or remissions from serious illnesses. One of their characteristics is indeed authenticity. But it is crucial to recognize that even when a person with cancer reduces her stress, clarifies her values, and changes her life, she still may not recover physically although her efforts are likely to extend life and dramatically increase happiness.

Like Shirley, Julia has also been asking questions about how satisfied she is with her life, not because she has an illness, but because these kinds of questions are integral to the midlife transition she is experiencing at forty-four. Was writing all those papers that she despised in order to get tenure and move up the academic ladder worth the personal sacrifice? The constant political wrangling at her college is disheartening, and since Julia is in a strong position to be promoted to departmental chairperson, a great deal of time is taken up with petty collegial infighting and posturing. Is it worth staying in academia with all the backbiting and competition? Couldn't she do just as much good in the world, and get even more satisfaction by being a clinical social worker rather than an academic? Julia is in the process of re-visioning her life to be consistent with the values triad. How can she have the best relationships with others, enabling her to give and receive love? What will lead to a reduction in stress and a sense of serenity? How can she be of service in a way that feels personally creative and enlivening?

THE MIDLIFE TRANSITION

Some people might think that Julia's intense questioning, and her final decision to leave academia on the verge of becoming departmental chairperson, means that she is having a midlife crisis. In this scenario she would be depicted as a desperate woman, longing for her younger years, who is likely to commit rash acts that she later comes to regret. But do droves of women in their forties really get sucked into patterns of anxious rumination, depression, affairs, or the compulsive purchase of cruise tickets and snappy red sports cars? Reading popular magazines would lead one to believe that menopausal women, in particular, go berserk prior to entering deep depressions and can be resurrected only by face-lifts, tummy tucks, and hormone replacement therapy.

The concept of the midlife crisis, which is usually attributed to psychologist Daniel Levinson, is, he says, prone to be grossly misunderstood. Levinson has described several periods of transition in the course of the life cycle during which we evaluate what has come before and what lies ahead, changing our lives dramatically in the wake of that examination. One of these periods occurs between the ages of forty and forty-five, when we reflect back upon the culminating life structure of early adulthood and set about constructing an entry life structure for middle adulthood.

This period of transition, while it involves considerable reflection, is not necessarily a crisis. It is a developmental stage rather than a psychological emergency and for emotionally healthy women it is not a time of crazed acting out, driven by fears of being over the hill. It is a time of calculated, rational action. For some women, however, the normal stress that occurs during the midlife transition does precipitate a psychological crisis either because unresolved problems from previous parts of the life cycle undermine their coping capacities, or unrelated major stresses similarly overwhelm their ability to cope. Midlifers, for example, are often called the sandwich generation. Women in their forties may not only have children to care for, but also aging parents. Since careers also tend to be in their most demanding stage, midlife can be a challenging time, and even reasonably well adjusted women may have periods of feeling "over the edge" when various life stressors conspire to make life temporarily unmanageable. To call this a midlife crisis, however, would be a misnomer. It would be a life crisis that just happens to be occurring during a woman's midlife transition.

Levinson conducted in-depth interviews with a small number of homemakers and career women in the midlife transition, between the ages of forty-two and forty-five. While the total number of interviews is too small to qualify as a random sample representative of all women, he did describe some interesting themes, all of which centered on relationship—to self, to family, and to work. As the children get older, and particularly when they leave home, a woman's relationship with her spouse comes into the forefront. What is the quality of their marriage? Has it changed from the time they set up housekeeping? Is it mutually encouraging? Is she willing to stay with it during the next season of her life? Her relationship to her job may also be changing. Rather than focusing on advancement, Levinson's sample talked of their preoccupation with the *meaning* of their work and whether or not it felt creative and enlivening to them as individuals.

Most of his homemaker sample told poignant stories that revolved around wishing to end their previous life structure of caretaking. They were tired of continually meeting the needs of husbands and children and yearned not only to be free of the burden of caring for others, but also to develop independent interests and capacities, to come into their own. Perhaps the most striking part of the homemaker interviews was how sad these women felt. They had upheld their end of the marriage bargain, caring for the home, the kids, and their husband. Many had also worked and helped the family financially. But rather than feeling fulfilled, most felt cheated, as if they had given their youth away to others and gotten very little love and comfort in return. Most of the homemakers told stories of being completely fed up with husbands who treated them like maids rather than desirable, interesting women. They missed romance and sex. They had dreams filled with sadness, anger, confusion, and the need to remake their lives in a way that centered on fulfilling themselves rather than giving themselves away to other people, who, it seems, gave very little back.

The thirteen women in Levinson's career woman sample represented a diverse group. Only two of the thirteen were living the dream of their entry-level life structure, which had been to balance career, marriage, and motherhood. The rest were either unmarried, childless, or had left their careers. These women were faced with constructing a new ideal for midlife. Like Julia, they began to realize that being a successful career woman was filled with compromises and trade-offs. Those in corporate positions also realized that discrimination against women increased in the upper echelons of company structure and that there was not just one "glass ceiling" to penetrate on the way to success.

At every level there were new obstacles. Many women became disgusted with the competitive nature of corporate life and began to focus on the inherent value of what they did, rather than the outer trappings of their job position. Levinson summed up the feelings of career women during their midlife transition, "Their great hope was that work would provide a stronger experience of creativity, satisfaction, and social contribution, that it would become more playful and loving rather than a matter of proving oneself in a highly competitive world."

THE PHYSIOLOGICAL METAMORPHOSIS OF MIDLIFE

Just as our values and outer life structures are undergoing a midlife metamorphosis, so are our bodies. The physiological changes that occur in a woman's forties prime her for the next stage of life, which is characterized by coming more fully into her creativity and making an expanded social contribution. Unfortunately, these physiological changes have been cast in a negative light that cause women to fear midlife rather than look forward to it. Perimenopausal women, who are leaving the childbearing years behind, need a new understanding of the very positive changes their bodies are undergoing, as do younger women who will come into midlife soon enough.

I consider menopause a second puberty, an initiation into what can be the most powerful, exciting, and fulfilling half of a woman's life. As adolescents we gain the physiological capacity to mother children. As midlife women we gain the capacity to mother the larger world, beyond the boundaries of our nuclear family. The years leading up to the first puberty, during which our bodies undergo a stunning metamorphosis in shape and function, are considered a positive time of change, an entrance into womanhood and the reproductive years. In contrast, the perimenopausal years, culminating in the second puberty of menopause, are considered a negative time of change because they herald the end of our reproductive years. While being freed from the fear of pregnancy has the potential to rejuvenate a woman's sex life, allowing her to become more sensuous than before, many women have equated the end of fertility with the end of sexuality.

Many years in clinical practice have convinced me of the fact that how we fare during the second puberty is largely a matter of attitude. Women who feel as if they are coming into their power are likely to have an increased interest in and appreciation of sex. They look vital and healthy, and they feel in the prime of their lives. Many of my patients commented that they felt as though they were becoming women, just entering their fullness, with the advent of midlife. In contrast, women who buy into the myth that menopause is the end of their womanhood, the beginning of a rapid decline into aging and loss of attractiveness, start to lose their vitality. They look and feel old. Research studies indicate that negative views of menopause also increase the number of unpleasant symptoms associated with the change of life including hot flashes, night sweats, fatigue, achiness, and sleep disturbances.

Negative feelings about menopause are a holdover from old beliefs that women are valuable only because of their ability to bear children, beliefs that are still held by the majority of the world's population. Although most Western women are outwardly liberated from this point of view, the liberation is very recent, and the idea that our major value resides in childbearing is still very much alive in the collective unconscious. This is why the Traditional Homemaker Figure still has so much control over our lives.

Any period of metamorphosis is challenging. During the time when a caterpillar is becoming a butterfly, it is neither one nor the other. It must endure a period of ambiguity, a time in a relative no-man's land, while it is changing. Perimenopausal women similarly reside in a body that is rapidly changing and can be strangely unfamiliar. Vivid, prescient dreams and hot flashes can be disconcerting. Author Gail Sheehy writes in her excellent book on menopause, *The Silent Passage*, that "It is during perimenopause—in their forties—that women feel most estranged from their bodies. The important thing to know is that for two or three years the female body is out of synch with its own chemistry." The attitude we have toward these "out of synch" years makes all the difference to how we experience body, mind, and spirit during the several-year period that eventually culminates in the cessation of menstruation—the actual menopause. Just what are the chaotic signs of a changing body?

My friend Carolina Clarke was sitting in our living room one evening when she was in her midforties. Her eyes bulged wide as she suddenly clasped both hands to her breasts, which felt as though they were on fire. Five years later, now that her menses have stopped, Carolina recognizes "the night of the flaming breasts" as the herald of perimenopause. During the next four years she noticed hot flashes, mood swings, and wildly irregular periods, which eventually stopped. After six months, just when she thought that she had entered menopause, her menses returned as a raging tide—the familiar phenomenon of flooding that occurs when the lining of the womb becomes progressively thicker when periods are skipped, finally shedding as a copious flow that Carolina dubbed "the Red Sea." Once she had crossed the sea, a few cycles later, her menses stopped for good, an event in which we can place some confidence only after a full year has passed since the last menstrual flow.

The physical concomitants of the perimenopause vary greatly from woman to woman. Some have no recognizable outer manifestations of "the change" until one day their periods simply stop. Others report a dizzying array of experiences. In the positive mental column women report an increase in the vividness of dreams, experiences of déjà vu, the recognition of synchronicities, an increased confidence in their judgment, and stronger intuition. Many also report the kind of fierce, cut-through-it-all wisdom that helps break old patterns and fuels the move toward authenticity that both Shirley and Julia experienced. In the negative mental column some women report an inability to focus on what's happening outwardly (probably because we're meant to go through a period of inward focusing) and mood swings. In the physical column women report a wide range of symptoms that vary from few to many, from positive to negative, and from mild to strong. These include either fatigue or vastly increased energy, body aches, sore breasts, migraine headaches near the end of the menstrual period, bloating, longer or shorter cycles, occasional heavy bleeding (flooding) and/or progressively lighter bleeding, hot flashes, night sweats, and either an increase or a decrease in sexual interest.

I was forty-seven when a friend gave me a book on natural and hormone-replacement approaches to menopause, a subject that we will discuss in the next chapter. I immediately thought, "Hey, I don't need this, my period still comes like clockwork." Like many women, I thought of menopause as an all-or-nothing event like catching a cold.

Either you had it or you didn't. I was nearly fifty before I experienced obvious physical signs of perimenopause including rare night sweats, a very occasional hot flash, headaches during menstruation, and periods of fatigue and muscle aches that, on the first few occasions, I thought were the flu. But as I reflected back on my earlier forties, obvious changes were occurring in my dream life, personality, and intuitive access to wisdom that are the most important, and generally overlooked, aspect of the change of life.

The average woman completes the metamorphosis of perimenopause and emerges into the postmenopausal years when she is 48.4 years of age. Part of the physiological shift she undergoes is a decline in the female hormones, estrogen and progesterone, and a corresponding increase in the production of male hormones. A woman's testosterone levels, for example, increase twentyfold by the advent of menopause, which relates to the emergent fierceness of what I call Guardian archetype. During the metamorphosis, women who were passive gradually grow more assertive and our vision begins to expand beyond the small realm of friends and family to the realm of humanity at large. Carl Jung wrote, quite rightly, that we awaken to social responsibility sometime in our forties. This need to guard the circle of life, and to protect our fragile earth and its occupants from exploitation, is related to the physiological shift that occurs during midlife.

THE EMERGENCE OF THE INNER MALE

Jung theorized that at midlife women begin to develop their male side, or *animus*, while men begin to develop their feminine aspect, or *anima*. In an essay on the stages of life Jung wrote of a case reported in the ethnological literature about a midlife Indian warrior chief to whom the Great Spirit appeared in a dream. "The spirit announced to him that from then on he must sit among the women and children, wear women's clothes, and eat the food of women. He obeyed the dream without suffering a loss in prestige. This vision is a true expression of the psychic revolution of life's noon, of the beginning of life's decline. Man's values, and even his body, do tend to change into their opposite." The tendency of older women to grow hair on their faces, and of older men to develop breasts and padded bellies are, like it or not, part of this reconciliation of opposites.

During the midlife metamorphosis I had a dream about my emerging male aspect that I entitled "Iron Joan." It actually took place in an iron foundry. In the dream, the world's men were being systematically murdered by women because they had brought the world to the brink of destruction through greed and profligate use of natural resources. I was running from the foundry with my husband, whom I was trying to protect, having given him my name tag. Since I was obviously a woman, I was safe. I managed to rush him into a car, drive him to a friend's home, and hide him in a spare room. The friend had a daughter who looked quite odd; she had a full beard that covered her entire body. I was marveling that my friend acted so normally toward this strange child, until I realized that she, too, was a bearded lady.

As I thought about this vivid dream, it seemed to reflect the problem I was having in claiming my masculine side. Like many women, I fear the aspect of maleness that is associated with power and aggressiveness, which, when misused, can indeed destroy the world. For that reason, prior to the dream, my male aspect had been carefully hidden away. In fact, I overcompensated on the female side by going to great lengths to put on a mask of self-effacing sweetness so that no one could accuse me of being aggressive, or even wanting to succeed. And if they did, I became extremely defensive and then found a way to nurture someone as a form of penance, a way of affirming the feminine.

In the dream, I believe that my husband represented my own male aspect. The women trying to murder him represented not only myself, but the collective unconscious of all women who fear expression of their animus. Nonetheless, this part of myself was precious, so I went to great lengths to protect it. I had to step into my male aspect by orchestrating a daring escape from the foundry and providing safe haven for my husband. These behaviors represent the nurturing use of male energy. Finally, I was confronted by the bearded girl child, a representation of my own budding inner wholeness—the integration of male and female. At first I pitied her until I recognized that her mother, an extremely successful scientist and businesswoman whom I very much admire, accepted her daughter completely because she herself was a bearded woman. The message was clear to me. It was time to accept the beauty and rightness of my animus so that I, too, could become whole. I discovered strength and courage in an iron foundry, a place of power where raw ore undergoes a change into steel. This is the transformation that occurs physiologically for every woman at midlife, but which she must consciously embrace.

I like to think of hot flashes as the power source for the iron foundry in which an expanded feminine power is being forged through developing and accepting our male aspect. While hot flashes are often attributed to estrogen deficiency, and estrogen does indeed relieve them, research indicates that women with severe hot flashes actually have estrogen levels equivalent to women who don't have any hot flashes at all. And although estrogen is often perceived as the fountain of youth, and its decline the inevitable herald of aging, the peri- and postmenopausal elevation of the hormones FSH and LH, which *rise* up to 1,300-fold, are usually ignored.

REWIRED FOR INTUITION?

During the years that we ovulate, the pituitary gland releases a pulse of FSH and LH at midcycle, just before ovulation. FSH stimulates the release of the egg, and LH causes the sac of cells that once surrounded the ovum to convert into a temporary endocrine (hormone-producing) organ, the corpus luteum, that manufactures progesterone. When ovulation stops at menopause, the body does a seemingly odd thing. Rather than decreasing FSH and LH, the pituitary pumps out more, to try, so the theory goes, to goose the spent ovary into coughing up a few more eggs. When no eggs appear, and the body fails to produce the estrogen and progesterone that once signaled the pituitary to stop secreting FSH and LH, even more of these hormones are released. The question remains as to why the body, which preserves amino acids—the building blocks of proteins—would waste those that go into making FSH and LH, along with the energy necessary to synthesize these hormones long after the egg supply is exhausted. Our bodies are naturally geared to conserve energy and protein, making the most of the natural resources we take in through food. Most likely these hormones have a purpose after menopause that is different from what it was before, and that purpose has not yet been discovered.

Gynecologist Christiane Northrup, author of the excellent book *Women's Bodies, Women's Wisdom*, has advanced an interesting theory based on the postmenopausal rise in LH and FSH. Premenopausally, LH and FSH are high only near ovulation. Therefore, our brain levels of these hormones wax and wane in an alternating fashion, depending on where we are in the menstrual cycle. Postmenopausally they are high all the time, and since there is some preliminary evidence suggesting that FSH and LH may act as neurotransmitters, Dr. Northrup hypothesizes that these neuropeptides may eventually turn out to be the "hormones of wisdom," an actual mechanism through which women's nervous systems are rewired at menopause to become more intuitive.

The implications of this theory, which has yet to be scientifically proven, are intriguing. Does the rise in FSH and LH that occurs at ovulation in our reproductive years correlate with the increased receptivity to vivid dreams and intuitive impressions that many women report at that time? If so, the dramatic increase in these hormones post-menopausally would favor continuous receptivity to intuitive impressions on a daily basis, rather than just for a few days around ovulation each month. Naturopathic physician Farida Sharan believes, on the basis of her clinical impressions, that women's menstrual cycles produce a kind of alternating current of intuition premenopausally that is changed into a direct current postmenopausally. Herbalist Susan Weed makes the point that all over the world men are sitting in prayer and meditation trying to reach the intuitive state of interdependence that menopausal women are in naturally.

In a wide diversity of ancient cultures, from Native American to Middle Eastern, from African to aboriginal, and from European to Icelandic, postmenopausal women are prized for their intuitive wisdom and ability to gain knowledge for the good of the society through dreams. In many of these cultures, women who had reached the age where they "retained their wise blood," an archaic understanding of menopause, were trained as oracles, priestesses, shamans, and healers. In the seventeenth century, Christian writers still insisted that old women were filled with magic power because their menstrual blood remained in their veins. Modern society has lost an appreciation of the special value of postmenopausal women, whose clarity, vision, and fierceness are potentially great gifts to society.

THE BIRTH OF THE GUARDIAN

My friend Rima Lurie was celebrating her forty-eighth birthday in our sleepy little mountain town of Gold Hill. Several of her women friends, most of us in our late forties, gathered around the window seat of her beautiful stone home, built from rocks gathered from the surrounding meadows and heated entirely by sun and wood. Before building her solar home, which fits perfectly into the landscape, Rima had lived on the land for more than ten years in an old settler's cabin with wood heat, but no electricity or running water. Years of listening to the silence, studying the light, the trees, the seasons, the winds, and the many animals who are drawn to her sanctuary informed the building of a home in which she could live self-sufficiently as part of the delicate but wild mountain ecosystem. We were basking in the rose-colored radiance of the late afternoon sun, gazing out at the snow-capped mountains of the Continental Divide, when Annie—another strong, self-sufficient, and gentle mountain woman—started an interesting discussion about perimenopause and the metamorphosis in both body and attitude that it represents.

We shared the "symptoms" of this gradual metamorphosis, which ranged from hot flashes to muscle aches and migraines; from oddities in sleep patterns to night sweats and personality changes. But those latter changes were far different than the medi-hype (men's medical opinions about women) that focuses on moodiness, grumpiness, and whiny moaning about the passage of our youth. They centered instead on a kind of passionate protectiveness, an unwillingness to let even small injustices pass unchallenged. Annie, who not only cuts her own wood, but fells and drags the logs, mused on her newfound response to the sightseers who rubberneck their way down the mountain road, oblivious to the fact that "locals" depend on it for getting into Boulder. "When they don't move over after a friendly honk," she shared, "I have visions of shooting out their kneecaps." This brought knowing smiles and chuckles from the rest of us, previously the most self-effacing, friendly group of healers, hospice workers, and nurturers you could hope to meet.

The summary of our discussion was that we were coming into a time of life where there is no time for nonsense and no tolerance for self-centered people who disregard the rights and needs of others. Levinson documented this growing fierceness as it evolves from a woman's early twenties into her midlife transition. In our younger years, we are more likely to compromise and put up with situations that are undesirable. For instance, many homemakers in Levinson's sample lived in poor marriages, in a state of "psychological divorce" during their twenties and thirties. When the strong midlife realization dawned that they had spent their lives giving to other people and getting very little back, many of the women developed a fierce, steadfast resolve to take back their lives and their power. No longer willing to put up with bad marriages, three women involved in his study divorced at about this time.

I have observed both in my clinical practice and amongst my large cadre of midlife friends that even previously mild-mannered women develop a kind of fiery directness during the midlife metamorphosis that can cut in both directions. When a woman is emotionally mature and psychologically healthy this new boldness is channeled into personal, family, and social causes that further the feminine values of relationality and interdependence. When a woman is emotionally immature, however, her fierceness may express itself instead as increased self-hatred, fear of aging, or an unfortunate need to control other people.

Those of us who have accomplished enough of our personal healing to reach emotional maturity by the end of the first half of life, enter the second half with a remarkable burst of new energy, a protectiveness both of our own rights and those of others. For this reason, I have chosen to call the midlife woman the Guardian. Perceiving injustices, and willing to call people and institutions to their higher purposes and best expressions, the woman who steps fully into the Guardian archetype has the ability to encourage the best in herself and others. As she continues to develop a larger social, political, and spiritual perspective throughout her forties and fifties, she is prepared to become a visionary with the heart and guts to create change.

The number of women now entering midlife is an unprecedented historic event that I firmly believe is sowing the seeds for a cultural reawakening of feminine values. Mark Gerzon wrote a wonderful book on midlife called *Coming into Our Own*. In it he comments that the time we think of as midlife seems to recede as we come up to it, quoting a conversation that aging Katharine Hepburn and Henry Fonda have in the memorable movie, *On Golden Pond*. When Hepburn talks about having dinner with another midlife couple, Fonda growls that they're not in midlife—after all, people don't live to be 150 years old! But the average woman already lives to be 75, and if she's in good health at 65, statistically she can expect to live until 84. So, if your health habits are reasonable and your genetics and destiny conspire for longevity, at 42 you have about half your life left to live, as good an estimate of midlife as we can make.

The ranks of midlife women are now swelling dramatically, a fact that is obvious to anyone observing how advertisements pander to the majority. Suddenly the ranks of lithe Generation X models are being swelled by real, honest-to-God, sumptuous midlifers who have meat on their bones and money in their pockets. A local Denver women's book club is now in hot demand by the media, having starred in a homey, successful commercial touting the benefits of alpha-hydroxy skin cream. I was born in 1945, just before the baby boom, which technically began in 1946. Would-be fathers came home from World War II and mothers (at least some of them) retired from war jobs in banks, offices, and munitions factories to become the June Cleavers of the 1950s—the last generation of women who were raised in the tradition of the feminine mystique to conform to a single role—that of homemaker. Those of us who are now in our forties and early fifties are their daughters, a hinge generation with opportunities for work and self-expression that most of our mothers did not have.

Women "baby boomers" are an enormous, and increasingly vocal, group of strong, self-sufficient, knowledgeable, and emotionally mature women. Furthermore, it is estimated that the number of women between forty-five and fifty-four will increase by one half (from 13 to 19 million) by the year 2000. Our time has finally come; midlife is actually what's happening sociologically. As we encourage one another in embracing the promise of midlife, we have the historic opportunity to create and implement visions that can change our troubled society for the better. Margaret Mead talked about the midlife years as a time when women came into "postmenopausal zest." Using that God-given energy together we can usher in much-needed change in the coming millennium and restore feminine values based on interdependence and respect for life.

MIDLIFE OPPORTUNITY: ENERGY AND EMPTYING

Naturopathic physician and herbalist Farida Sharan is one of my interesting mountain neighbors. She wrote a marvelous book, *Creative Menopause*, which contains a compendium of natural alternatives for those interesting midlife years when the body is readjusting its physiology, and we are undergoing a truly remarkable metamorphosis that aids substantially in the move toward authenticity. She writes, "Women are essentially receptive in nature. For our first thirty-five to forty years we take the world into our being. Many women reach a saturation point around menopause where we cannot take in any more. We have to clear. We have to empty. We have to find our essence again."

I kicked off the midlife cycle of emptying by going through my closets and giving away three quarters of my clothing. I was like a woman possessed. If I hadn't worn it in a year, or had anything but the warmest feelings for a piece of clothing, out it went. My sisters-in-law, who were the recipients of the closet-emptying ritual, were thrilled. I have not replaced most of what I gave away. It's amazing how many different outfits a few pieces of great clothing can be combined into. I dress much more creatively than I used to because by pruning the forest I can now see the trees. It takes less energy to decide what to wear when there are fewer choices, and energy is of the essence. Why be drained by things that are meant to serve us or to create comfort or enjoyment?

How many people are drained by credit-card payments for things that they didn't really need? In 1996 it was reported that the average American making twenty-five thousand dollars a year carried a staggering twenty thousand dollars in credit-card debt. What about the American dream of two cars in the garage? After totaling up the real costs, not only in dollars but in other kinds of energy, my husband and I decided to make do with one car instead of two, even though it is occasionally inconvenient. The freedom from servicing, inspecting, washing, repairing, insuring, and paying for a second vehicle more than makes up for the times that we have to invent creative transportation solutions. Whenever I see something in a store that attracts me, an inner voice asks the question, "What are you willing to give up for that?" If it will take time, care, or money best saved for retirement, it stays where it is.

Living lightly is a way to loosen the hold of the world and keep one's energy for better purposes. It is also a way to honor the reality that our planet's resources are limited, and that material possessions are part of a vast interdependent network that involves the need for more fossil fuels, the cutting down of the rain forests, the exploitation of Third World labor and the continuing destruction of the environment. Fewer cars on the roads, fewer clothes in our closets, fewer nonessentials translate into a cleaner environment for us and for future generations.

Many women comment that midlife brings an emptying in the area of friendships as well. People who are consistently negative use up both time and precious energy. Whereas earlier in life many of us had a hard time saying no to people and things that were draining, the rising energy of our own masculine aspect makes saying no much easier in midlife. As the ovaries begin to make less estrogen and more androgens (male hormones), we figuratively develop the hormonal balls to set our boundaries and decline invitations that do not feel nourishing. What is the real cost of "going to lunch" with a person you'd rather not see? When we empty out those commitments, friends, and belongings that do not support the midlife values triad of love, serenity, and service, we reclaim energy that can be used for better purposes.

By midlife our emotional skin ideally begins to thicken as well. The psychologically healthy woman in her forties has become capable of letting go of small hurts, rather than hanging on and nursing them into energy-draining grudges. Years of observation and experience bring the realization that people often speak or act thoughtlessly, whether out of ignorance or out of their own woundedness. We have an important energetic choice to make when that happens. We can either take on their problems and give up our own freedom, peace, and energy, or we can let little hurts go, maintaining our integrity. The conundrum of adolescence, "How can I get my own needs met without being selfish?" is one that we revisit at midlife with much more experience and testosterone under our belts. It becomes clear that meeting our own needs is not selfish, but sane, since continuing to place other people first may not only rob them of their own challenges to growth, but drain our own energy to the point where we become depressed or ill.

THE GIFTS OF THE MIDLIFE TRANSITION

A friend of mine, nurse/researcher Janet Quinn, defined the midlife gifts of authenticity, emptying, and rededication to the feminine values in a very concise way. When I asked Janet what was true, what was authentic, she replied, "It's a felt sense more than anything else. Integrity. Being of one self; body, mind, and spirit. Where being and doing are integral. Where action flows from values, from what has most meaning rather than from trying to make things all right. Acting out of your inner integrity and not out of expectations and cultural norms and definitions of what is right, wrong, good, bad, successful or unsuccessful. If you can sit in the possibility of emptying and metamorphosis it's exquisitely freeing—for the first time I have the freedom to become who I am because I don't fear other people's judgment or my own. This has dropped into the background, the foreground has continued to be, 'In the moment is this true for me?'

"It doesn't matter what other people think although relationship matters immensely. The desire is to be in relationships where the truth is spoken with care, with compassion. So you act with awareness of others, but are free from what-would-the-dean-think? kind of stuff. People's feelings are very important to me. This is not about selfishness—that seems like an important difference. It's about self-ness, being self-full, soul-full, trusting yourself deeply enough to know that if your commitment is to act with integrity you will by definition relate with care, compassion, and love, so that you don't have to be afraid that by being yourself you won't care for others.

"That's the essential process, and there are no guarantees. If you do all your work well and get clear and strip all these things away you still may not walk into forever and live happily ever after. Next week I could get cancer or be hit by a truck or lose my house. There's no guarantee from the cosmic lifestyle underwriters. You can't slip under the radar and avoid what life might offer by doing things right. I want to think, 'Hey, I've done all the work, I'm standing here naked, now I get all the rewards.' Well, guess what? Maybe, but there's no guarantee."

I laughed with delight at Janet's profound wisdom about the lack of cosmic underwriters. People are always looking for ten steps to permanent abundance and perfect health. But there aren't any. We learned that from the biblical story of Job. You can do everything right and still suffer. Janet commented that when you live from integrity, empty of expectations, "the outcome is almost irrelevant—it's the moment-by-moment process that counts." This realization, and the freedom that it brings, are great gifts.

The physiological metamorphosis of menopause is another special gift that supports authenticity and self-fullness. The relative increase in testosterone levels during the perimenopause helps women to use their male aspect with authority, developing the passion and confidence that allow us to stand up for what we think is right. The rewiring of our nervous systems to become direct currents of intuition enables us to access wisdom greater than our individual knowledge and to become conduits for a higher wisdom that helps us remember the original instructions of spirit, the way that human beings can live in balance and harmony.

The great Lakota medicine man Mathew King summarized the simple instructions for happiness and morality given to human beings by the Great Spirit, "Our instructions are very simple—to respect the Earth and each other, to respect life itself. . . . Respect is our Law, respect for God's creation, for all living beings of this Earth, for our mother the Earth herself." The midlife woman, who has spent half a lifetime developing her basic gifts of relationality, has a natural spiritual appreciation of these instructions. Furthermore, she has the power and the voice to bring the message of respect, care, and interdependence to all people and help rekindle a reawakening to these core feminine values throughout society. It's no mistake that the current movement of psychospiritual healing is composed largely of women in their thirties, forties, and fifties. We are awakening en masse and beginning to deliver a much-needed message of health, hope, and healing to the world.

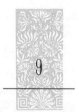

AGES 49–56: FROM HERBS TO HRT

A MINDFUL APPROACH TO MENOPAUSE

In September of 1995, over eleven hundred physicians, researchers, psychologists, healers, and interested women from fifty countries gathered in San Francisco for a meeting of the newly formed North American Menopause Society. It was founded in response to the need of both health-care providers and women to understand this critical period of growth and metamorphosis. While the prevalent attitude about menopause is negative for most Americans, papers presented at the meeting showed that women in other cultures viewed menopause more positively. A study at the prestigious Karolinska Institute in Stockholm, for example, found that menopause was a time of increased self-esteem for many Swedish women, as it is in many indigenous cultures. In cultures that celebrate menopause women suffer fewer "negative" symptoms. What can this teach us about the feminine bio-psycho-spiritual feedback loop? Are certain foods and vegetables consumed in other cultures, but generally lacking in the Western diet, integral to making a smooth menopausal metamorphosis? Is hormone replacement therapy (HRT) really a fountain of youth that relieves symptoms during the time of the change and prevents osteoporosis and heart disease later in life? What of its side effects? In this chapter we will review both natural and pharmaceutical approaches to menopause and the inherent values and possible pitfalls of both.

THE RISE OF COMPLEMENTARY MEDICINE

At fifty, parts of Julia's story bear a striking resemblance to my own life, and we merge for a time. She is vitally interested in menopause research for personal as well as professional reasons. Still a striking woman, the once-virgin landscape of her face bears witness to a full life. Laugh lines run like little rivers alongside her mouth; tiny creases radiate from the corners of her eyes, testimony to joys and sorrows deeply felt; a slight looseness of the skin beneath her chin lends a subtle softness to the whole. Still menstruating regularly, she is beginning to have some hot flashes, and is concerned about the possibility of osteoporosis later in life since her mother, Sylvia, who is close to eighty, has lost several inches in height and developed a fairly pronounced dowager's hump.

Increasingly, Julia's medical social work practice is filled with midlife women, a testimony both to the fact that this sector of the population is increasing rapidly, and to the fact that women are more likely to ask for help coping with medical and psychological problems than are men. The hypothetical Boston hospital where Julia works has taken seriously the 1993 study of Harvard physician David Eisenberg, in which he found that one third of the American public had visited providers of alternative medical care in the year 1990, and set up a clinic for alternative approaches to women's health concerns, including PMS and menopause. Julia runs this clinic in partnership with a woman gynecologist by the name of Sophie Garrett.

Eisenberg and his colleagues surveyed the use of sixteen types of alternative medicine ranging from acupuncture to massage; from chiropractics to meditation, and found that more people had consulted an alternative practitioner than had visited a primary practice physician in 1990. The fact that nearly fourteen billion dollars had been spent, close to twelve billion out of patients' own pockets rather than from insurance, sent a strong message to physicians, researchers, and hospitals. Many hospitals nationwide have decided that since Americans are using alternative medicine, often without informing their doctors, that it is time for orthodox, or allopathic, medicine, to take notice of the phenomenon and enter cooperative alliances with alternative practitioners. Furthermore, half of all medical schools now offer courses in alternative therapies. Books like *Spontaneous Healing* by physician Andrew Weil, who majored in botany while an undergraduate at Harvard, and makes a compelling case for following a natural route to health based on diet, exercise, attitude, correct breathing, and relaxation skills are best-sellers. While Dr. Weil generally writes prescriptions for herbs, rather than for pharmaceuticals, he finds himself in the same position we do in this chapter. When it comes to weighing the effects of HRT on cardiovascular disease and osteoporosis, the jury is still out and the choice between alternative and orthodox approaches is one that each woman and her physician must carefully consider together.

The term *alternative medicine* is generally used interchangeably with *complementary medicine.* I personally prefer the latter term since studies indicate that the great majority of people do not use treatments like acupuncture, massage, herbs, visualization, meditation, or dietary therapy to the exclusion of allopathic medicine, but rather to supplement it. Complementary approaches, in general, are based on bringing the body back into homeostasis, or balance, so that the healing mechanisms of the body can function as nature intended. Approaches like homeopathy, acupuncture, polarity therapy, Reiki healing and Jin Shin Jyitsu, which are based on energy medicine, are predicated on the understanding intrinsic to traditional Chinese and Ayurvedic (Indian) medicine that the body is enlivened by a life-force energy, which, when blocked or weakened, can predispose a person to illness or uncomfortable physical symptoms. Like a radio with spent batteries, a human body with low levels of this energy performs poorly. Treatments that increase the energy flow can therefore sometimes be curative, and in other instances, set the stage for allopathic treatments to work better.

MINDING THE MENOPAUSE

I have had the pleasure of working with a large number of peri- and postmenopausal women who attended the ten-week mind/body clinic for stress-related disorders that I directed during the 1980s, and I have continued working with women in a variety of weekend retreat settings since that time. Although our hospital program was not intended to relieve menopausal symptoms, many women reported that headaches, anxiety, depression, mood swings, and hot flashes improved as a result of the program. Some women commented that hot flashes decreased in number and that they could also dramatically reduce the duration and intensity of hot flashes using belly (diaphragmatic) breathing. This simple technique involves taking one deep cleansing breath, like a sigh of relief, and then imagining that you can breathe directly into the belly. Feeling the belly expand with the inhalation and flatten with the exhalation, you can count ten on the first in-and-out breath, nine on the second, all the way down to one. This controlled breathing elicits the relaxation response and short cuts the fight-or-flight response. Heart rate and blood pressure decrease, the mind calms, and even hot flashes begin to dissipate.

My clinical observations have been confirmed and extended in several studies. One of my former students, psychologist Alice Domar, coauthor of the book *Healing Mind, Healthy Woman*, and director of the women's health programs at Harvard Medical School's Division of Behavioral Medicine, collaborated with psychologist Judy Irvin on a study of controlled relaxation for hot flashes. They studied thirty-three women ranging from forty-four to sixty-six years of age, whose periods had stopped for a minimum of six months, and who experienced at least five hot flashes daily. The women were divided into three groups; two control groups and one who learned to elicit the relaxation response and did so daily for seven weeks using a twenty-minute prerecorded audiotape. The relaxation-response group reported a significant decrease in the intensity of hot flashes (28 percent), anxiety, tension, and depression, while the two control groups showed no significant changes. While the relaxation-response group also reported fewer hot flashes, the group size was so small that the change was not what scientists call statistically significant. In other words, though it was highly suggestive, it could have been due to chance. The authors believe that with a larger group of women, significant reduction in hot-flash incidence would also have been observed, a result that has been reported by three other research groups who showed reductions in hot-flash frequency of 40, 60 or 70 percent with simple forms of relaxation training including belly breathing and progressive muscle relaxation.

Physical exercise may also influence the frequency of postmenopausal hot flashes. A group of researchers in Scandinavia found that "moderate and severe" hot flashes, sweating, heavy breathing, and palpitations were only half as likely to occur in women who rated themselves physically active as opposed to those who were sedentary. Physical exercise produces a myriad of metabolic and hormonal changes that may affect hot flashes, and it is also a strong stress reducer. Stress itself has been shown to make hot flashes worse. A report in the *Journal of Health Physiology* was based on laboratory monitoring of twenty-one postmenopausal women who reported frequent hot flashes. The women experienced significantly more hot flashes during lab sessions when they were subjected to psychological stress than in a nonstress session.

A woman's response to stress, and her ability to maintain her serenity, are obviously important factors in the experience of hot flashes. So is her attitude about the hot flashes. British psychologist Frances Reynold of Brunel University College tested the hypothesis that negative feelings might make hot flashes worse. She recruited fifty-six women, none of whom felt that they had any control over when or if a hot flash might occur, although some did recognize that they could control their feelings about them. Those women who were embarrassed by the hot flashes, or who had thoughts about being over the hill and unattractive, reported significantly more distress than women who took them in stride.

Two researchers at Guys Medical Hospital School in London decided to see if changing women's attitudes toward hot flashes might reduce their frequency or severity. They recruited twenty-four women who had complained about menopausal symptoms to their physicians. The women got to choose hormone replacement therapy, simple monitoring, or a psychological training group. Some women went into the training group right away and others were enrolled after a waiting period to control for the placebo effect—in other words if they expected the group meetings to help then they might have gotten better simply in anticipation. The women in the training group went to four one-hour classes over a six- to eight-week period in which they learned deep breathing and relaxation techniques, and a "cognitive component" that centered on becoming aware of and changing negative feelings about the symptoms. Women who were monitored or in the waiting period for the training did not improve. But those who took the four classes had 50 percent fewer hot flashes. Three months later over 90 percent of the women in the training group reported significant improvement and a quarter of them had no more hot flashes at all.

REFRAMING HOT FLASHES AS PSYCHOSPIRITUAL OPPORTUNITIES

What if hot flashes were a psychological and spiritual opportunity rather than a bothersome symptom? According to the research this positive point of view should decrease the number and severity of hot flashes, so let me tell you an interesting story. At the age of forty-seven, a spunky Frenchwoman by the name of Alexandra David-Neel left her privileged, protected life. Leaving her husband behind in Paris, she shaved her head, dressed in saffron and crimson robes, traveled halfway around the world to the forbidden mountains of Tibet, and sneaked into a monastery by impersonating a male lama. She was, in fact, an archetype for the Yentl that Barbra Streisand made famous in her movie about an Orthodox Jewish woman who gained entrance into an all-male yeshiva in a similar way. David-Neel was one of the first Westerners to witness ancient Tibetan sacred rituals, and to learn personally the meditation practices.

During the full moon one February she attended a ritual in which monks stripped naked in the freezing temperatures of a Himalayan cave, wrapped themselves in wet sheets and proceeded to dry them when their bodies liberated prodigious amounts of heat during a meditation practice called *tumo yoga*. The monk who dried the most sheets was considered the highest adept. *Tumo* means "fierce woman" in Tibetan. It refers to the life-force energy of every human being (regardless of gender) that circulates in thousands of small channels called *nadis*, similar to the acupuncture meridians. Seven energy reservoirs called *chakras* determine the distribution and flow of this bodily current, and physicians from Chinese, Ayurvedic, and many other traditions heal disease and foster health by balancing and freeing blockages in this vital electricity that they believe enlivens every cell and organ.

Tumo yoga was practiced primarily for spiritual reasons, however, rather than for physical healing. Through a series of meticulous visualizations and the repetition of sacred sounds, the monks raised the life-force energy through the lower energy centers up to the highest chakra at the crown of the head. In the process, they believe that they are burning away mistakes, erroneous beliefs, and ego attachments that keep them from fully recognizing the nature of their True Self, which in Tibetan is called the *rigpa*, and which we might recognize as our "best self"—or essence. Dr. Herbert Benson, a physician who has done a great deal to elucidate the physiology of diverse meditation practices, traveled with a team of scientists to northern India, where the Tibetan community lives in exile, to study lamas practicing tumo. Benson and his team found that, indeed, these monks could raise their surface temperatures more than ten degrees Fahrenheit during the meditation practice.

Perhaps there was no need to go to India. Benson could simply have studied women having hot flashes. What if women used hot flashes in the same way that the monks did, consciously thinking of their stresses and worries and offering them to be burned up in the inner fires of transformation. When I have a hot flash, for example, I think of what has been stressful for me lately. Am I exhausted from traveling, tired of writing, or worried about my children? I say a little prayer of thanksgiving for all the good things in my life, and then I offer the specific things that are stressing me to the inner spiritual fire of the hot flash in much the same way that people talk of giving up their troubles to God.

I believe that hot flashes represent a rising and rebalancing of the life-force energy that can help women burn off stress, rather than adding to it, an idea that has some basis in Chinese medicine. During the perimenopausal years the Chinese believe that there is an increase in the active, dry, hot element called *yang* energy. Before thirty-five a woman is more *yin* (moist, receptive, passive) but during the change of life her yang begins to express itself. She becomes more passionate about ideas, quicker to anger, faster to defend herself or others. As more "hot" yang energy begins to move through the acupuncture meridians, at first the flow is kind of jerky as we get accustomed to using the new energy. Those jerky manifestations of rising yang give rise to hot flashes. But as the meridians open to the yang energy and we get used to using it, so the theory goes, the flow stabilizes.

According to the forty-nine different cultural traditions that base their medicine on life-force energy, when we have a lot of stress, either through poor diet and lack of exercise, or because of poor coping skills, the life-force energy can't flow smoothly through the meridians. In that case the flow of energy would have a hard time stabilizing and hot flashes would persist. All the research we reviewed on the reduction of hot flashes through stress management, breathing, and meditation exercises that are supposed to increase the flow of life-force energy makes perfect sense from an energetic standpoint.

How do you view hot flashes? Naturopath and herbalist Farida Sharan writes of her approach to her six months of hot flashes, which was one of intense self-observation, in her highly recommended book, *Creative Menopause*. Looking forward to each episode, she experienced the energy as beautiful, even ecstatic, although they sometimes brought up painful memories that needed to be cleared up through reflection, forgiveness, or the taking of some specific action. She writes, "Toward the fourth month the releases increased in purity, beauty and intensity. As I grounded more deeply in my being, I began to perceive the reality of my life around me in a different way. My martyr persona was dissolving. I could no longer do things the way that I always had. I saw more deeply. It was as though I read people's minds and motives and looked at my life and realized that I would have to change." Farida's description of the dissolution of a habitual way of relating to the world is typical of the process of emptying and coming to authenticity that we discussed in the last chapter.

Now that we have had a chance to review the effect of attitude, belief and stress on one manifestation of menopause, hot flashes, let's follow the progress of "Cynthia," a woman who is about to participate in the alternative menopause clinic that Julia and gynecologist Sophie Garrett have started, as she uses her symptoms as an impetus to make major changes in her thinking and lifestyle. She will be our guide through the maze of potential mind/body, pharmaceutical, and natural approaches to menopause that confront today's woman.

A TYPICAL CASE HISTORY

At fifty-two, Cynthia is still menstruating, but irregularly. She occasionally skips periods, sometimes has periods barely two weeks apart, and occasionally she has very heavy bleeding, or flooding. Several times daily she has hot flashes that last for two to three minutes, turning her face and neck crimson and leaving her with an odd tingling sensation, but these are not as disturbing as night sweats that cause her to throw off damp covers and often strip off her nightgown. No sooner does she fall asleep, it seems, that she awakens chilled and puts her nightgown back on, only to wake up a short time later hot and sweaty. The cycle often repeats itself two or three times in the course of a night, and she sometimes wakes up for good at four or four-thirty A.M., unable to doze off again.

Like many people whose sleep is interrupted, Cynthia suffers from two kinds of fatigue. One stems from simple lack of sleep. The other has its roots in what she calls the "three-A.M. horror show." In the quiet hours of the night, she finds herself at the mercy of an anxious mind that seizes on potential problems and embroiders them into catastrophic proportions. Her mind goes round and round considering the what-ifs. What if her daughter Susan can't raise the money to go back to school to become an X-ray technician? What if her husband's company downsizes and he loses his job? What if her college-age son drinks too much and gets in an accident? What if the breast pain she has been experiencing means that she has breast cancer?

Her nightly worry fests are increasing her stress level. As a result she is fatigued during the day and experiencing more hot flashes than she would if she could relax. Furthermore, she finds herself drawn to her typical "stress diet" including plenty of sweet rolls, coffee, diet soda, and fatty meat, her traditional comfort foods. The sweets, often eaten instead of a meal, are causing major fluctuations in blood sugar, leading to hypoglycemia and fatigue. The caffeine is increasing blood pressure and heart rate, making her hot flashes worse. More caffeine is present in the diet soda, as are phosphates, which displace calcium from her bones, predisposing her to osteoporosis. Furthermore, the caffeine is contributing to the fibrocystic condition of Cynthia's breasts, causing mastodynia, or breast pain. The bacon and hamburgers she loves have four strikes against them. They are high in fat, contributing to the possibility of heart disease. They are high in protein, and unlike excess carbohydrates which the body stores as fat, excess protein is excreted through the kidneys, pulling calcium along with it and adding a further risk factor for osteoporosis. They contain nitrates, which are potent carcinogens, or cancer-causing agents. Fatty meats are also high in a type of fat-soluble chemical pollutant called xenoestrogens. Residues of organochlorine pesticides that are used to spray crops, xenoestrogens concentrate in animal fat. Butter, for example, has a 2,000 percent greater concentration of these pollutants than the grain fed to the cows. While research is still in its preliminary phases, several studies have indicated a relation between xenoestrogens—which work like estrogen in the body—and the development of breast cancer.

In her initial hour-long interview with Dr. Garrett, Cynthia is counseled to change her diet drastically. Eliminating or at least greatly cutting down on caffeine, substituting six or seven glasses of still water (carbonated water is high in phosphates, which drain minerals) for diet sodas, getting most of her protein from beans and tofu rather than meat, increasing whole grains, fruits, and vegetables (green, leafy vegetables are a particularly rich source of calcium), and cutting back on sweets are the main recommendations. Not only will these foods decrease the risk of several types of cancer, heart disease and osteoporosis, they will also reduce stress. Cynthia is also counseled to try 600–800 IU of vitamin E daily, which often helps reduce hot flashes, as well as four grams of vitamin C, 1,000 mg of calcium citrate, and 400 mg of magnesium for her bones, and a natural, high-potency vitamin B tablet.

Cynthia wonders whether she needs tranquilizers to help cope with her anxieties. Maybe sleeping pills would help, too, she ventures. But Dr. Garrett assures her that the coping and relaxation skills she will learn in the menopause program, coupled with the dietary changes, are likely to be all that is needed. Cynthia then discusses her hopes and fears concerning hormone replacement therapy (HRT) with estrogen and progestin. Some of her friends are on HRT and seem to be thriving. Furthermore, her mother has osteoporosis, so does that mean she'll get it, too, without estrogen replacement? But her mother has also had breast cancer, which makes Cynthia a poor candidate for estrogen or HRT. Are there any natural hormonal alternatives?

Cynthia confides to Dr. Garrett that some her friends started on HRT with high hopes, and ended up going off it a few months or a few years later because they didn't like the side effects. One friend felt as though the hormones were making her crazy. She felt premenstrual all the time—tense, anxious, bloated, and with extremely sore breasts. Another got terrible headaches and ended up on two other drugs to control them. The headache remedies made her tired and after six months she threw out both the hormones and the other drugs and visited a Dr. Chen down in Chinatown. Now, Cynthia says, this friend takes an herb called *dong quai*, chews ginseng root, and has started doing tai chi. Dr. Chen also prescribed acupuncture treatments. Her friend looks ten years younger, is full of energy and says that she hasn't felt better for years. Cynthia wants to know what Dr. Garrett thinks about these alternative treatments.

After a complete physical, which included low-dose X-ray bone-density measurements (dual-energy X-ray absorptiometry, or DEXA) and levels of follicular stimulating hormone (FSH) and luteinizing hormone (LH), Dr. Garrett discussed her findings with Cynthia at a second hour-long meeting. She didn't bother to measure estrogen levels because, although estrogen does show cyclic variations throughout the menstrual cycle, and although absolute levels decrease by 40 to 60 percent after menopause, daily levels are highly variable. A one-day measurement, therefore, is of little value. Cynthia's FSH and LH were high, as they are during perimenopause and early menopause, and her bone density proved to be in the high normal range.

During the five or so years that comprise the perimenopause, women lose 2–5 percent of their bone mass each year, after which their bones stabilize. Because Cynthia doesn't smoke and has walked regularly for years, her bone mass is good to begin with, a fact that makes an enormous difference as the perimenopause progresses. Studies indicate that 50 percent of the bone loss experienced over a woman's lifespan actually occurs *before* menopause begins, and thus is unrelated to a decrease in estrogen production. The woman at greatest risk for osteoporosis is likely to be the one whose prior health habits have contributed to bone loss since she was an adolescent. Cynthia's mother, for example, is a smoker who has never exercised. She'll drive around the block three times to get a parking space half a block closer to where she's going, and has an impressive diet cola habit. Since carbonated beverages leach minerals from the skeleton, as does smoking, and since she lacks the exercise that helps deposit calcium in bones, her mother has multiple risk factors for osteoporosis. Other risk factors include estrogen and progesterone deficiency, as well as a family history of osteoporosis, never having had a child, heavy alcohol use, a high-fat, high-protein diet, and a diet low in calcium and magnesium.

Cynthia and her doctor are both relieved at her excellent bone density measurements. Were they very low, Dr. Garrett might have started Cynthia either on a low-dose natural progesterone cream or a natural estrogen (both are derived from yam roots) which in her experience causes far fewer side effects than Premarin, which is derived from the urine of pregnant mares and contains seventeen different types of estrogen, most of which are not native to human beings. Furthermore, Premarin is produced under intensely inhumane conditions. Pregnant mares are permanently catheterized and confined to a tiny space. After they give birth, they are allowed to nurse their foals for only one week so that they can be impregnated again as soon as possible. These living Premarin factories often die during their second or third pregnancy from the stress of confinement. Some women who have decided to try hormone replacement insist on using either synthetic estrogens or natural phytoestrogens, out of compassion for the horses.

Three major classes of estrogen—estrone (E1), estradiol (E2), and estriol (E3), are synthesized by the human body. Both estrone and estradiol have been implicated in breast cancer, while there is impressive evidence that estriol might even be protective in this regard. While a discussion of the potentially protective effects of estriol are beyond the scope of this book, Christiane Northrup, M.D. provides a full discussion of research, and a listing of pharmaceutical sources through which physicians can order estriol derived from natural, vegetable sources in her excellent book, *Women's Bodies, Women's Wisdom.*

The use of phytoestrogens, derived from plant sources, is relatively new. On the minus side, it takes larger doses of estriol to produce the same effects that estradiol and estrone yield, so that some doctors combine small amounts of the latter hormones with the estriol. On the plus side, estriol is natural and used in its native form by large numbers of women worldwide since it is particularly prevalent in soy products. Anthropologist Michelle Locke of McGill University in Montreal reported that Japanese women experience far fewer hot flashes and night sweats than American women, which she attributes to a diet rich in soy-based foods like tofu and miso, which are high in phytoestrogens. So Cynthia and her doctor discuss whether bean-curd burgers sautéed in tamari or HRT are likelier to be the better bet for her. They also discuss a third option, which is gaining considerable attention in the alternative medical community, the use of natural progesterone cream instead of estrogen supplementation, as we will discuss below.

IS MENOPAUSE ACTUALLY AN ESTROGEN DEFICIENCY?

The orthodox medical view is that menopausal symptoms are caused by estrogen deficiency. But how good is the evidence that has made Premarin a pharmaceutical superstar and convinced many physicians that HRT is the best way to prevent heart disease and osteoporosis as well as to alleviate negative menopausal symptoms? And if HRT is so effective at reducing these symptoms, why do so many women discontinue it because of side effects ranging from depression and mood swings to weight gain, fluid retention, and high blood pressure that seem worse than their original complaints? Furthermore, what of the increased risk of stroke, or breast and ovarian cancer linked to HRT?

HRT hit the mainstream in January of 1964 when *Newsweek* published an article entitled "No More Menopause," based on the work of New York gynecologist Robert A. Wilson. Wilson subsequently authored a book entitled *Feminine Forever* that touted estrogen therapy as a fountain of youth that would prevent women from experiencing the "tragedy" of menopause, which would leave them dried up, sexless, and depressed. In the wake of this publicity, doctors were leafleted by drug companies selling estrogens, and women eager to be "feminine forever" became willing guinea pigs for the first wave of hormone replacement therapy.

Soon enough, estrogen replacement therapy (ERT) was found to cause precancerous or cancerous changes in the uterine lining of nearly a third of the women taking it. The reason is that estrogen stimulates cell division, including cells in the uterine lining, breasts, and ovaries. The risk of uterine cancer was soon overcome by adding synthetic progestins (since natural progesterone cannot be patented there is no profit in it for drug companies), which resulted in a menstrual period each month in which any damaged uterine lining cells could be shed. ERT had become HRT, at least for women who still had an intact uterus.

Some male physicians have suggested that women might as well have hysterectomies (removal of the uterus) and ovariectomies (removal of the ovaries) at menopause, since these organs are potential sites of cancer. A professor of pathology who lectured us at Harvard Medical School in the 1960s went one step further. Why not remove both breasts at the same time, he suggested, and also relieve women of the possibility of developing breast cancer? The same ridiculous reasoning, of course, would suggest that men should be castrated and have their prostate glands removed as soon as they've sired all the children they want. Even after menopause, the ovaries continue to secrete hormones, and there is evidence that removal of the ovaries prior to menopause may increase the risk of heart disease. Following hysterectomy some women also report decreased sexual responsiveness.

There are times when hysterectomy and/or ovariectomy can be life-saving as in the case of cancer, or necessary to relieve severe pain and bleeding caused by extensive fibroid tumors or widespread endometriosis. Approximately six hundred thousand women each year have hysterectomies, and Dr. Stanley West, chief of reproductive endocrinology and infertility at St. Vincent's Hospital in New York has estimated that five hundred thousand are unnecessary. Following a complete hysterectomy (which includes the ovaries), a woman is thrown into an immediate surgical menopause and HRT is usually required for life. If your doctor recommends a hysterectomy, it is essential to get a second opinion.

What about the data linking HRT to breast cancer? In 1995, the results of the largest study to date were published in the prestigious *New England Journal of Medicine*. Postmenopausal women using HRT for five or more years have a 30–40 percent greater risk of developing breast cancer than do women who do not use hormones. On the other hand, HRT users have a 29 percent reduction in colon cancer risk. HRT has also been linked with an increase in the risk of ovarian cancer, which is particularly alarming since this disease is difficult to detect until it is relatively far advanced. Implicated in a variety of other health problems, ranging from asthma to high blood pressure, HRT is hardly a choice to be taken lightly. In fact, a 1995 study in the *American Journal of Respiratory and Critical Care Medicine* reported that women on HRT were 50 percent more likely to develop adult-onset asthma than those who did not take hormones. The negative aspects of HRT are usually dismissed by its proponents with the argument that since more women die from heart disease than breast or ovarian cancer, and since HRT protects against osteoporosis and colon cancer, a woman is still better off with HRT in the long run, unless she has a family history of breast cancer. But how good is the research on which this what-would-you-rather-die-from argument rests?

Osteoporosis, or the progressive loss of bone mass, is a preventable specter that haunts women as they age. The lifetime risk of an osteoporosis-related fracture is 40 percent, and fragile, easily fractured bones are a significant cause of pain, disability, depression, and loss of the will to live. As my mother aged I feared that she would fall and break a hip, ending up in a nursing home since half of all women with hip fractures never walk again. And 20 percent of women with broken hips die within a year of their fracture. But is estrogen a panacea? Estrogen does increase bone mass by inhibiting the function of osteoclasts, little Pac-Man-like cells that eat old bone so that new bone can be laid down. Our bones remodel throughout life in accord with how we bear weight, and how we exercise. For example, when the orthodontist applies braces to straighten teeth, the braces put pressure on the bone that holds the teeth in place. Osteoclasts respond to this pressure by eating away the bone on the far side of the tooth, giving it room to move. Osteoblasts lay down new bone on the near side of the tooth to hold it in place.

While estrogen decreases osteoclast activity, thus increasing bone mass, it has no effect on osteoblast activity. In other words, it doesn't build new bone. On the other hand, exercise does increase osteoblast activity, as does progesterone. Over the next few years, research should be able to provide evidence as to whether estrogen-and-progesterone combinations or progesterone alone are best for the prevention and treatment of osteoporosis. And in the meantime, remember that most bone is lost before menopause even begins. A low-fat, low-protein diet rich in fiber and green leafy vegetables, regular exercise, and the avoidance of smoking, alcohol, and carbonated beverages whose high phosphate level displaces calcium from bones is the best strategy for maintaining healthy bones throughout the life cycle.

The data on estrogen and heart disease should also be evaluated with an eye to prevention. The major risk factors for heart disease are a sedentary lifestyle, a high-fat diet, cigarette smoking, diabetes, high blood pressure, and stress. The stress factor, actually, may be of greater importance than any other. One study found that the majority of first heart attacks were not related to any of the five common biological risk factors listed above. They occurred on Mondays between eight and nine A.M. and were related to the stress of job dissatisfaction. So, to view women's heart disease as a result of estrogen deficiency is an oversimplification of a complex problem. Like osteoporosis, heart disease begins to develop well before menopause and is related to a multitude of risk factors. And while many studies indicate that estrogen helps reduce heart disease deaths in postmenopausal women, some other very significant studies do not. Let's review a few vital statistics before we look at the data.

Heart disease is the major cause of death for both men and women in the United States. Every year 40,000 women die of breast cancer, while 250,000 die from a heart attack, and an equal number die from diseases of the heart and blood vessels. These statistics are a shock to many women who fear breast cancer but may not give a second thought to heart disease. Furthermore, heart attacks are more lethal for women than men. A woman is twice as likely to die from a heart attack than a man is (the mortality rate is 50 percent for a woman, 25 percent for a man) and twice as likely to have a second heart attack. Since heart disease develops about ten years later in women than in men, and risk begins to increase postmenopausally, low estrogen levels have long been considered a risk factor. Premenopausally, women have higher levels of HDLs (good cholesterol), and lower levels of LDLs (bad cholesterol) than do men. After menopause, a woman's total cholesterol level increases, HDLs drop and LDLs rise. Since estrogen plays an important role in lipid metabolism, it seems to follow that it might prevent cardiovascular disease postmenopausally. But the data are mixed, as well as being confounded by the fact that synthetic progestins like Provera are often included along with estrogen in HRT, making it impossible to tell if the progestins or the estrogen were the cause of any changes in blood lipids or heart disease risk.

One of the most famous studies of cardiovascular disease is the Framingham Study, an ongoing epidemiologic study that has generated a large series of papers dating from the early 1980s. This well-regarded study showed no reduction in coronary artery disease as a result of estrogen replacement. Furthermore, postmenopausal women taking estrogen had a 50 percent increase in the risk for stroke. A study that is purported to show a significant effect of estrogen on the prevention of cardiovascular disease is the Nurses' Questionnaire Study, based on statistics gathered from over 48,000 nurses. An article published in the *New England Journal of Medicine* in 1991 indicated that risk of death from heart disease was 39 percent less in nurses currently using hormones and 17 percent less for former hormones users compared to nonusers. In an excellent critique of this study, physician John Lee makes the point that the hormone users were also less likely to have diabetes, less likely to smoke, and more likely to exercise. In other words, they had a lower general risk for heart disease. Lee concludes his critique with an even more compelling fact. During the study, only 2.6 percent of the nurses died (0.2 percent of the entire sample) and only 8.9 percent of the total of 112 deaths were from heart disease. To calculate risk on this basis would be equivalent to observing 500 nurses until one finally died from heart disease, much too small a sample to uphold the argument that estrogen prevented heart disease. Furthermore, as in the Framingham Study, there was a significant increase in strokes among hormone users.

THE ROLE OF PROGESTERONE IN MENOPAUSE

Dr. John Lee, who critiqued the Nurses' Questionnaire Study, also questions the medically prevalent hypothesis that bothersome menopausal symptoms are a reflection of estrogen deficiency. Instead, he hypothesizes that the primary problem is one of progesterone deficiency, leading to a relative *excess* of estrogen. His work is extremely controversial, but worthy of further research. This is a basic sketch of his argument. First of all, women continue to produce estrogen throughout life, at levels that approximate 40–60 percent of the amount that they produced in their twenties. Progesterone production, in contrast, often drops to levels lower than in men after menopause. Medical research has focused almost entirely on estrogen, however, neglecting the fact that progesterone has a variety of important functions beyond that of thickening the uterine lining to receive a pregnancy during the childbearing years.

Among other functions it stimulates bone growth and is a natural diuretic and antidepressant. In addition, progesterone opposes some the effects of estrogen. For example, estrogen causes release of the stress hormone, cortisol, while progesterone neutralizes it; estrogen leads to water retention while progesterone is a diuretic. The ratio between the two hormones is critical for the maintenance of homeostasis, or biochemical balance.

Research that is summarized in Lee's provocative book, *What Your Doctor May Not Tell You about Menopause*, suggests that menopausal symptoms, osteoporosis, and heart disease may not be due to estrogen deficiency, but to a *relative estrogen excess*, due to progesterone deficiency. The synthetic progestins, like Provera, that are included in most HRT prescriptions do not have the same biological effects as natural progesterone and can create a host of side effects including fluid retention, depression, breast tenderness, cervical erosions, jaundice, blood clotting, and stroke. Natural progesterone, on the other hand, has no known side effects. It is also not patentable and therefore of little interest to drug companies, but has been found helpful in shrinking fibroids and alleviating PMS, hot flashes, and other menopausal problems, as well as preventing and treating osteoporosis. And unlike estrogen, its benefits do not seem to be outweighed by risks.

During our reproductive years, many menstrual cycles are anovulatory, that is, the ovaries fail to produce an egg. When there is no ovulation, the corpus luteum, which normally grows from the follicle or egg sac that once housed the ovum, cannot form. Since the corpus luteum produces progesterone, anovulatory cycles result in low progesterone relative to estrogen. These are the cycles accompanied by breast tenderness, decreased sex drive, depression, bloating, weight gain, headaches, and foggy thinking that Lee cites as symptoms of relative estrogen excess. During the perimenopause, progressively more cycles become anovulatory. The best treatment, according to Lee, is the use of low-dose natural progesterone cream, which is applied for the last two weeks of the cycle to areas where the skin is thin, such as the face, breasts, inner arms, backs of the knees, inner thighs, neck, or belly. The progesterone is absorbed into the subcutaneous fat and then released into the bloodstream. Such creams, which are available at many health food stores, vary widely in progesterone concentration. Some have effectively none and others provide 20 to 30 mg in an average daily application of a half teaspoon to a teaspoon. Lee's book contains an index, and ordering information for creams with appropriate progesterine concentrations. For some women, the cream may be an effective treatment for hot flashes, bloating, depression, headaches, and other symptoms that Lee believes are due to relative estrogen excess. Using X-ray bone density measurements, he has also found that progesterone is very effective in building new bone and treating osteoporosis. Nonetheless, relatively few large-scale studies on natural progesterone have been carried out.

Considering the bewildering array of possible treatments, it is of utmost importance to find a physician who is willing to work as your partner. Without question, some women thrive on HRT and find that their quality of life deteriorates without it. Despite the risks, HRT is probably worthwhile for them. But the most conservative approach to managing the menopause is to expose yourself to the least possible hormonal risk. If your bone density measurements are low, for example, and your physician is willing to help you experiment, you might decide to make appropriate changes in diet and exercise, use natural progesterone cream, and see if bone density increases. If it does not, then natural estrogens can be tried, reserving Premarin as the last line of treatment since it is high in estradiol and increases cancer risk, unless your doctor can make a compelling argument for its immediate use.

A MIDLIFE MEDITATION EXERCISE

You might enjoy this meditation exercise, which will not only help to elicit the relaxation response and reduce stress, but also help you reframe your attitude about menopause. Based on the research we have reviewed, and my clinical experience, it may also help reduce hot flashes and other unpleasant symptoms ranging from insomnia to anxiety. Meditation in any form also produces what has been called a "flow" state, in which the practitioner becomes more observant of the inner flow of images, ideas, and sensations that underlie intuition and creativity. Ideally, you might practice this entire meditation once a day for a week, and then just steps two, three, and four for the next three weeks. At the end of the twenty-eight-day cycle, assess whether it has had a positive impact on you. Needless to say, meditation is not a replacement for a thorough medical evaluation or for any medication that your physician may have prescribed. If, however, you do notice positive benefits, you and your physician may together decide on a revised approach to any treatment you might require for menopausal symptoms.

You might wish to record this meditation to play back to yourself, with or without pleasant music in the background. If you do so, pause at the dots (.....) and be sure to allow sufficient time to complete each part of the process. You can also order a prerecorded version, which I narrate, from Mind/Body Health Sciences, Inc., whose address and phone number can be found in the Appendix at the back of the book. Side one of the tape is the complete meditation and imagery process. Side two is a meditation based on steps one through four of the exercise.

- Step One: Find a quiet place where you will not be disturbed by other people, animals, or the telephone. Plan to spend twenty minutes by yourself.

- Step Two: Sit or lie down in a comfortable position, covering yourself with a blanket or quilt if the room is cool. Close your eyes and begin to focus on the flow of your breathing.....You might notice that your body expands gently on the in breath.....and relaxes down on the out breath.....(Continue for a minute or so.)

- Step Three: Imagine that the breath is your life-force energy or *chi*. You might even experience it as light that enters your body just below the navel, then moves into your chest, and is finally drawn up into your forehead.....Then follow the breath out from forehead, to chest, to belly.....The breath is like a wave of energy, filling you.....belly, heart, forehead.....allow any stress to empty in the reverse direction.....from forehead, heart, and finally from the belly.....Continue to feel the way that the *chi* moves into your body like a wave.....and the way that tension leaves as the wave recedes. (Continue the *chi* breathing for another minute or two, or in the case of using just steps one through four, continue for another ten to fifteen minutes.)

- Step Four: As the *chi* fills your body, and the tension leaves, notice or imagine that your entire body is beginning to feel pleasantly and comfortably warm, as if glowing with an inner light. Affirm for yourself, "The energy of my body is coming into perfect balance. I am whole, healthy, vibrant, and creative."

- Step Five: Imagine now that your body of light is lifting out of your physical body and traveling to a sacred grove of trees that surrounds a quiet pond. Take a moment and let your imagination fill in the scene.....Notice the way that the sunlight and shadow play on the leaves and on the water.....Are there any sounds?.....Birds, or frogs.....wind or music?.....There is a rustle of leaves and a woman, somewhat older than yourself, yet somehow ageless, enters the grove. She may be a biblical figure like Mary or Sarah.....or perhaps she embodies the energies of a goddess, angel, or higher teacher.....or perhaps she is a contemporary woman whom you deeply admire.....You sit down together on a fallen log and she takes your hands and looks into your eyes, explaining that she has been waiting for you all your life, waiting for this sacred midlife passage during which you are coming fully into your feminine power.....this time in which your male and female energies are coming into a new balance. She asks you to take a moment and focus inward on the energy currents that are flowing in your body.....You feel the deep peace and receptivity of your feminine nature as a deep pool of wisdom and interrelatedness.....for a moment you drop your boundaries and become one with the earth.....the sky.....the wind.....the crickets.....the wise and powerful woman teacher.....then you begin to feel the passion and purpose of your male energy rising, enlivening you.....She asks gently if there is any old pattern of thinking or be-havior that prevents you from living from your highest vision.....She asks you to feel how that old pattern affects the flow of your en-ergy.....your peacefulness and your passion..... She then places her hands on top of your head and blesses you. You feel her wisdom and compassion as a flow of light and energy that moves down through your body, washing you clean of negativity and old patterns. The light from her hands continues to wash you clean, scrubbing the boundaries of your heart, which begins to glow and radiate blessings of peace to all beings.....

- Step Six: Thank this wise woman and imagine now that your body of light is returning to your physical body.....Rest in the peacefulness of an open heart until you are ready to come back and open your eyes.

THE GIFTS OF A MINDFUL MENOPAUSE

Cynthia's menopausal symptoms led to a reevaluation of her health habits and methods of coping with stress, which was a gift of health and vitality for her to carry into the subsequent cycles of life. She found that eating a low-fat, high-fiber diet gave her more energy than the fatty fare she had always loved, and also alleviated a nearly lifelong obsession with dieting. Rather than going on a diet that left her hungry and inevitably failed when she'd regain whatever weight she lost a few months later, changing her diet allowed her to eat a wide variety of tasty foods while gradually losing weight until she finally stabilized about ten pounds above her all-time college low. Since body fat is one of the primary sites where estrogen is synthesized after menopause, the average woman needs to be a little heavier than she was as a young girl, while avoiding obesity, which is associated with the development of heart disease, diabetes, and breast cancer.

While she'd heard of meditation, Cynthia had never been interested in trying it before. Since learning of its positive effects on stress, and be-cause it alleviated her hot flashes and night sweats, she was motivated to keep up a daily practice of fifteen to twenty minutes each morning.

Furthermore, she found that meditation decreased her anxiety and gave her a mental tool to deal with worry. Whenever she began to obsess about problems that hadn't occurred, like whether her husband's company might be downsized, she realized that while she had no control over the future, she did have control over the present. Right now, she could be grateful he was working. So she reframed her worry into gratitude, and bolstered the psychological shift with a physiological one by taking ten belly breaths, which moved her body chemistry out of the stress mode into the relaxation response.

Never before had Cynthia felt so good about herself, so fit psychologically and physically. More attuned to her body through meditation and the observation of the effects of her diet on her mood and physiology, she developed a kind of inner biofeedback mechanism that constantly alerted her to how different stimuli—ranging from a fight with her husband to a glass of wine—affected her energy. As she gradually became used to having more energy than she had had for years, Cynthia became conscientious about guarding that energy and the feelings of well-being and peacefulness that accompanied it. Never a heavy drinker, she gave up alcohol altogether because it left her feeling exhausted and flushed. A lifelong exerciser, she added a few minutes of hatha yoga to her walking routine because it energized her as well as stretching out her muscles. No longer a victim of "shoulds" about her health—eating a certain way or exercising because she knew it was the right thing to do—she became appreciative of how good her new health habits made her feel. She pursued them because she wanted to, not because she thought she should.

As Cynthia began to become more conscious of her body, mind, and energy, she found it easier to assert herself—knowing what lifted her up and what dragged her down. The clarity she was developing about herself made her more insightful about other people and situations. Almost unconsciously, her relationships began to change when she found ways to give people energy, rather than drain it. A word of encouragement, a kind look, and at times an honest assessment of a friend's situation that required Cynthia to say things that she once would have been uncomfortable about became matter of course.

The same penchant for honesty, and heartfelt concern about harmful situations and institutions, fed her desire to become more socially and politically active. When Cynthia's friend Margaret was diagnosed with breast cancer, for example, Cynthia responded by wondering why there was such an increase in this disease. Was it a result of diets too high in fat or chemical pollutants stored in fat? Cynthia formed a women's health caucus in her town, and they began to press their legislators for more research funds in women's health. The fierce and direct energy of the Guardian was beginning to rise.

Like Cynthia, we all can use the challenges of the menopausal metamorphosis as motivators to enter a new relationship with our bodies, minds, and energy systems. The gift of this middle cycle of midlife can be a vital and healthy lifestyle that not only helps protect us against many of the degenerative diseases that accompany aging, but also gives us the energy to use our wisdom to make this world a better place.

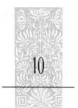

AGES 56–63: THE HEART OF A WOMAN

FEMININE POWER AND SOCIAL ACTION

At sixty, Julia, whose dark hair had turned prematurely gray in her forties, could be described as handsome, one of those women who has aged in a way that has rendered her even more beautiful than when she was young. She is trim and muscular, the result of long years of biking along the Charles River and hiking the mountains of New Hampshire many weekends. She wears her hair short, setting off her fine features with a pair of signature silver earrings that she almost always wears.

She is now the grandmother of Amanda's three-year-old daughter, Julia, named in her honor. She is also grandmother to four-year-old Jorge, and one-year-old Simon, the sons of Benjamin and his wife, Anna, whom he met in Mexico while he was a cruise ship steward. Miraculously, it seems, both her children's families have settled in the Los Angeles area, and while they live across the country from her home in Boston, at least the children are near one another. Furthermore, family visits are festive occasions, since they can all gather in Los Angeles at the same time, often with Julia's mother, Sylvia, who is now in her mideighties and the only living great-grandparent that the three little ones have known. Julia's father, John, died suddenly of a heart attack when Jorge was six months old, and Roger's parents had both passed on several years before any of the grandchildren were born.

Julia and Roger speak to their children and grandchildren at least once a week, and visit three or four times a year, often with Sylvia, who also lives in the Boston area. In between, letters, postcards, and parcels help make them a familiar and continuing presence. In his early seventies, Roger is now practicing medicine part-time, at least in theory. As soon as he scaled back his general medical practice, he promptly filled in much of the time by donating several hours a week to a free clinic for Boston's homeless. Julia soon joined him in her capacity as a medical social worker, and the two now spend Tuesday and Thursday afternoons doing volunteer work.

Recently, Roger has been talking about selling their home in Boston, moving into a condominium that will require less upkeep, and possibly signing back on with the Peace Corps or other volunteer organization offering medical services in Third World countries. Julia, however, is of two minds. On the one hand she is excited about the prospect of going back to Bangladesh, or perhaps India or Nepal, where the poverty is crushing and the need is great. On the other hand, there's plenty of need right here in the United States where her elderly mother, children, and grandchildren live, and she doesn't want to be out of touch with them for long periods of time. After several months of inquiries with various agencies, Roger and Julia settle on a compromise. They will travel to a village in central India, several hours east of Bombay, and spend a year doing work very similar to what they were doing in Bangladesh when they met in the Peace Corps. Roger will provide medical services and Julia will help out in a women's clinic, giving out information both on birth control and infant care. Roger will return once to the United States for a month, about halfway through the year, and Julia will return twice, so that she'll be gone for only four months at a stretch.

The Empty-Nest Syndrome: Replacing Depression with Altruism

Although Julia's nest was empty by the time she was in her early fifties, she never suffered from what has been called the "empty-nest syndrome," one more myth that has haunted woman's lives by contributing to the fear that once the children are out on their own our useful life is finished. Like most mothers, Julia found that caring for her children was a lifelong occupation that didn't end when they set out on their own. When the day-to-day concerns of caring for them at home were over, she took her nurturing energy and used it in other ways—in the midlife women's clinic she cofounded and in her volunteer activities. When we use our life-force energy to help others, research shows, our own health and vitality are protected.

Sociologist Phyllis Moen and her colleagues at Cornell University conducted a thirty-year study of 427 wives and mothers from upstate New York. They found that women who had multiple roles, and therefore a large network of social connections, were healthier, and lived longer, than those who didn't. Multiple contacts with other people not only reduce isolation, which many studies have shown to be a health risk, but the authors also concluded that it raises self-esteem, which has a positive impact on health, as well as encouraging preventive health behaviors. In particular, they found that women who were members of volunteer organizations lived longer, healthier, happier lives.

One of the clearest correlates of longevity, in fact, is in helping others, which is also a natural psychological and spiritual extension of midlife wisdom. Carl Jung wrote that the late midlife years were a time when our energy naturally moved beyond the concerns of our nuclear family into a concern with the world family. While this message has been adequately received by many men, however, it is still a revelation to most women, who have been conditioned to believe that our greatest utility is in childbearing and child rearing. If we believe that our useful years are over when the children leave the nest, and begin to isolate ourselves, it is no wonder that our energy diminishes and depression sets in.

Women, in fact, are two to three times more likely to become depressed as are men, although there seems to be no innate biological reason for this difference. Furthermore, forty studies have found the same preponderance of depression in women in thirty different countries. While research provides no specific answer to why women are more depression prone, there are several theories. First, because of cultural conditioning, women have a harder time expressing anger than do men and are therefore sometimes less honest about their feelings. Since some forms of depression are thought to be related to keeping anger in—turning it against oneself—one would expect women therefore to be more depressed. Second, more than a third of all women are sexually or physically abused during childhood, infusing them with a sense of helplessness because they were unable to do anything to protect themselves. In experiments with both animals and humans, the inability to escape noxious circumstances like electric shock or loud noise generally produces two behavioral consequences. First, when faced with a new challenge, the individual is slow to respond and may simply endure discomfort, making little or no attempt to overcome it. Second, if a random act (like bumping into a lever to turn off a shock) terminates discomfort, an animal is unlikely to recognize that its own action had something to do with improving the situation. Thus, an individual who has been made helpless previously, unlike one who has not, is very slow to learn. While we can't speculate on the emotions of animals, helpless human beings initially experience anxiety during times of threat, then become depressed.

One of the most compelling behavioral models of depression is based on helplessness. If we feel unable to control the world around us, changing those things that impinge negatively on the quality of life, we soon lapse into self-blame, hopelessness, and become less able to appreciate our own strengths. This makes us less resilient in the face of stress and more likely to become depressed when faced with life challenges. A third theory for the preponderance of depression in females is that women have a greater sensitivity to problems in relationships than do men. Men are more likely to respond to problems in their marriages by "medicating" themselves with drugs or alcohol, which anesthetize them emotionally, or by engaging in distracting activities like sports or work. Women, in contrast, are more likely to become emotionally preoccupied with problems that may seem insoluble. Their feelings of helplessness then lead to depression. A fourth theory hypothesizes that women's tendency to depression begins at puberty when they become aware of their relative powerlessness in a male-dominated society. Fifth, social factors such as lower wages for similar work, an emphasis on physical beauty that is hard or impossible to realize, and lack of professional opportunities have been related to depression. With regard to midlife women with empty nests, it has been found that women with stressful lives who do not work are at greatest risk for depression.

During my years of clinical practice, I worked with hundreds of late midlife women. The ones most prone to the depression of an empty nest had three characteristics in common. First, they had defined themselves primarily as mothers and had gained most of their self-esteem from nurturing their children. Second, they had limited their involvement in the world primarily to the activities of their children, highly involved in their children's sports events, social affairs, and education. Third, they often had poor relationships with their husbands, who felt as if they had been excluded from their children's lives by a woman who "took over," and also felt that they had been displaced from their wife's affection by the kids. When the children left home, these women were left adrift. The keel of their emotional boat had been hauled up, and they didn't know how to use their talents and energies. Furthermore, without the buffer that the children's activities had provided, they were suddenly left to face the reality of a poor relationship with their mate.

Most of the midlife women I saw were not examples of the empty-nest syndrome. The majority felt a sense of freedom and excitement when the children left home, a new lease on life. But research shows that even those women who do suffer depression and feel cast adrift when the children leave are not likely to remain stuck in that state. In fact, this period of midlife depression and grief over the loss of her family is likely to lead to a period of reevaluation that delivers a woman to the next phase of life—a larger concern with the world family. "Sandy," a former patient of mine, is a case in point. She had literally made her four children the entire focus of her days, and was at a loss without the constant commotion of her children's friends in the house, and the endless tasks that she had relished. She missed their music, their energy, even the excitement that the inevitable problems of the teenage years can bring.

Sandy was morose and depressed when I first met her. Mourning her lost youth, and the only role she had ever known, she bought in to the myth that her productive life was over. She felt sad, worthless, fatigued, and self-critical. What Sandy needed to know was that when one phase of life ends, we undergo a period of renewal as the next cycle prepares to unfold. It is natural to feel anxious or blue in these periods of emptying, the don't-know times that recur periodically throughout the life span. One role has passed away and the next has not yet emerged.

While Sandy was moderately depressed, she was not suffering from a full-blown clinical depression. The latter has been compared to falling into a black hole with no way out. It is characterized by symptoms that may include lack of appetite or overeating, sleeplessness or too much sleep, feelings of intense worthlessness and guilt, obsessive worry, lack of interest in sex or other activities that are normally enjoyable, extreme fatigue, trouble concentrating, anxiety, hopelessness, and feelings that one would be better off dead. Serious depression is a true medical emergency. Without treatment about 30 percent of depressed people try to kill themselves and unfortunately 50 percent of those attempts are successful. If you or a loved one has five or more of the above symptoms for a period of two weeks or more (one of the symptoms must be loss of interest and pleasure), seek professional help. The combination of drug therapy plus psychotherapy is very successful in alleviating depression in most cases.

Sandy's depression responded to a combination of psychotherapy, which helped her rebuild her marriage and develop a better sense of self, and activities that were outer directed, specifically toward helping others. The first step was channeling her energy into volunteer work, which almost immediately gave her a sense of purpose and helped the depression to lift. Twelve-step programs like Alcoholics Anonymous often prescribe the same treatment for depression, counseling participants to "get off their duff" and go help someone else. It makes intuitive sense that shifting the focus from our own problems to helping others might help to alleviate depression. It also makes neuroanatomical sense. Imaging techniques like positron emission tomography (PET scans) have been used to study changes in the brain during depression. An area in the prefrontal lobe, called the anterior cingulate area, is part of a structure called the limbic loop. The limbic loop is involved in the emotional aspects of thinking and behavior, and has a particular relevance to depression. When depressed, a person is self-absorbed. Depressed mothers, for example, may show little or no interest in their children. Blood flow to the anterior cingulate area increases when we are occupied with processing internal emotional information, and this part of the brain becomes active. In depressed people it shows hyperactivity, resulting in obsessive rumination. But when we shift the focus away from ourselves to the outside world, different brain structures become activated. Physical activity, like walking or jogging, helps to create a more outward focus. Helping others through volunteer work or other altruistic avenues does much the same thing. It pulls us out of ourselves, stimulating outer-directed brain centers involved in language and motor activity.

Once Sandy's depression had lifted, she found a new sense of direction. She enjoyed helping other people and decided to do so professionally. While earning a degree in social work, she met an entire cadre of midlife women in the same program, and found an interested, interesting peer group of friends who were all dedicated to using their nurturing capabilities and accumulated life knowledge for the good of society. A few years after we met, Sandy confided that she had never been happier in her life. Indeed, for the majority of those women who initially experience their children's departures with anxiety and depression, research shows that within five to ten years they are much stronger and better adjusted than men of the same age.

In *The Fountain of Age*, Betty Friedan reflects on why women live an average of 7.8 years longer than men in our culture, and what social as well as physical factors may account for the difference. She writes, "Could the continual need to change, the continual beginnings and ends confronting women in their reproductive role have strengthened them for age? In fact, I found many studies indicating that women experiencing the most change and discontinuity were the most vital later in life." She cites a study of women transiting through the empty-nest years that divided them into two groups, "statics" or "constrictors," versus "expanders" or "shifters." Sandy exemplified the latter group, women who had shifted and expanded their roles, rather than the former who stayed at home in roles that had shrunk. Shifters, on the whole, are highly satisfied with their lives. In fact, the years after the children have left home are often the most fulfilling time of a woman's life. And since there are now more women than ever before in history at this stage of freedom, experience, and influence, we have the opportunity to become a prodigious force for social change, while at the same time buffering ourselves from isolation, increasing our resiliency and satisfaction, and protecting our health.

CULTURAL CREATIVES: SPREADING THE FEMININE MESSAGE OF RELATIONALITY AND INTERDEPENDENCE

By midlife, most women have come to an appreciation of the feminine values triad of love, the expression of self-in-relation through which two people help bring one another into an expanded state of creativity and happiness; the sense of serenity that comes from authenticity; and service, the recognition that we receive great satisfaction from giving because all things are interrelated and interdependent. This latter value translates into a concern for the environment and the preservation of the planet for future generations.

A 1996 study by sociologist Paul Ray identified feminine values as the core of a new social movement that involves 44 million, or 24 percent of all Americans, whom he calls Cultural Creatives, or CCs. This movement began to appear in the 1970s and is unusual because it involves substantially more people at its outset than has any other newly emergent societal sector. There are two subgroups of CCs, what Ray calls Core Cultural Creatives and Green Cultural Creatives. The Core CCs, who represent 20 million Americans, or 10.6 percent of the population, are "seriously concerned with psychology, spiritual life, self-actualization, self-expression; like the foreign and exotic (are xenophiles); are socially concerned; advocate "women's issues"; and are strong advocates of ecological sustainability. They tend to be leading-edge thinkers and creators. They tend to be upper-middle-class and their male-female ratio is 33:67, twice as many women as men." The Green CCs, who represent 24 million Americans, or 13 percent of the population, "have values centered on the environment and social concerns from a secular view, with average interest in spirituality, psychology or person-centered values. They appear to take their cues from the core CCs and tend to be middle class."

Ray identifies three major worldviews in American society: Traditionalists, Modernists, and Cultural Creatives. The Traditionalists, whose roots can be traced to medieval Europe, tend to be rural, racist, and antiforeigner. They yearn for a return to small-town, religious America as it existed from about 1890–1930, and number 56 million strong, or 29 percent of the population. Modernists, whose roots can be traced back about five hundred years to the end of the Renaissance, have values centered on economic concerns, military strength, science, technology, and intellectual pursuits. This group consists of two factions: fairly open-minded liberals and more reactionary conservatives. The Cultural Creatives are the newest group, tracing their roots back to the spiritual movements that grew out of the Renaissance, early nineteenth-century American Transcendentalists like Emerson and Thoreau, and the newer movements of transpersonal and humanistic psychology, ecology, and the women's movements, which all date from the 1960s or later.

The values of Cultural Creatives that Ray lists include an interest in ecological sustainability that goes beyond environmentalism to an appreciation of nature as sacred, a concern for global problems of population and pollution, the adoption of simpler lifestyles, and an interest in rebuilding neighborhoods and communities. The interest of CCs in women's issues includes concerns about violence in society and in the home against women and children, an emphasis on fostering caring relationships, and a concern for family. CCs are also vitally interested in alternative health care, spiritual growth, and the importance of the inner life. This latter interest, however, is far from self-centered. CCs are not dropouts hoping to attain self-realization through contemplation of their solitary navels. They are interested in collective well-being and service projects that can help rebuild communities. In short, they function on a level that appreciates interdependence more than independence. Their own happiness grows in part from improving collective well-being.

The values of Cultural Creatives translate into some interesting lifestyle preferences. CCs like to read and listen to the radio (especially

NPR and classical music stations) more than watching TV, which they believe has very little worth. They particularly resent children's television programming and appreciate what Ray calls "whole stories" about consumer products. A whole story tells us where something came from, how and by whom it was made, and where it will go when we're done with it. It is a story of interdependence that helps us decide whether a product is good for the planet as a whole. CCs, therefore, are also avid label readers and well-informed shoppers. They enjoy technological products, health and gourmet food, which they may like to experiment with in the kitchen, and appreciate real things rather than imitations—leather rather than vinyl, wood rather than plastic. They enjoy traditional items that have a story behind them and this often reflects the creative way in which they decorate their offices and living spaces. They prefer homes hidden from the road, with access to nature, rather than "showy" houses meant to advertise their square footage to the street.

Ray's thesis is that the Cultural Creatives represent the potential for a "new and distinctive social force," which he calls Integral Culture based on the fact that, for the first time in history, we are developing a true world culture that must respond to the needs of all people, not just those from wealthy and powerful countries. This new culture will be faced with balancing ecology and economy; fostering better global communication; reconnecting with nature; and synthesizing a diversity of world beliefs, religions, and traditions with respect. The fact that a quarter of the population has embraced the values required to create an Integral Culture in a mere twenty years is very encouraging. And the fact that women are the majority of this movement is hardly surprising. But Ray points out that the coming of an Integral Culture is not yet a given, there is still a tremendous amount of work to do before the feminine values of relationality and interdependence can create a new world culture.

Women's values are gradually beginning to shift the zeitgeist in this country, though, not just through political action, but through doing what women do naturally, relating to other women. This translates into dollars—and into a medium to spread the message—in the entertainment industry. Naomi Judd, who retired from the country music scene when chronic hepatitis threatened her life, has taken to wielding her considerable influence to promote healing and spirituality. Oprah Winfrey, with a daily audience of millions, has used her influence in a similar way and plans to continue it through producing films that inspire, encourage, and heal. Stories about people who meet challenges and overcome them, stories about people who mend broken relationships, and stories about people who find healing even in sickness and death—like the movie *Terms of Endearment*—starring Shirley MacLaine and Debra Winger are examples of this genre.

Women are the fastest-growing segment of frequent moviegoers, and also rent 60 percent of the videos, which bring in more than twice the money spent in movie theaters. And more and more low- to medium-budget films about relationship are cleaning up at the box office. Many young female stars like Demi Moore, Michelle Pfeiffer, Jodie Foster, Meg Ryan, Sharon Stone, and Winona Ryder are turning into directors or producers, and rather than spending multimillions on rock-'em sock-'em violence films, they are interested in producing films that enhance people's lives. A *Time* magazine article quoted Sarah Pillsbury, a Hollywood producer, on the new genre of women's films. "Women tend to honor and validate daily life and human transaction and recognize that within the mundane the miraculous often exists."

Many of the best films are inspiring precisely because they validate the intrinsic spirituality of relationship and the day by day search to become authentic. *Steel Magnolias*, a play and later a film about a group of women in a southern town, advanced its message of women's resilience, care, and honesty, in part through everyday conversations that the women had in a beauty salon. Midlife women are thoroughly engaged in the process of life evaluation, emptying, and moving toward authenticity. Since they also make up a larger percentage of book buyers and moviegoers, it is not surprising that the entertainment industry is cashing in on our interest in psychological growth and spirituality. Author Susan Cheever has some interesting reminiscences about turning fifty, a time, she says, when she stopped searching for who she was and began to "inhabit my own life." Writing in *Living Fit*, a magazine for midlife and older women, she said, "I began to identify less with Gloria Steinem's remark at her fiftieth birthday party—'Fifty is what forty used to be'—and more with her sister-feminist Jane O'Reilly, who said, 'Fifty is not a delayed forty. Let there be less marveling at our wonderful preservation and more respect for the maturity of our minds and spirit.'"

WE CAN MAKE A DIFFERENCE, ONE BY ONE

We are not all meant to produce a movie or lead a movement, but each of us can look deeply within our hearts and listen for the voice of clarity and compassion that directs us in the daily acts of kindness and encouragement that comprise our essential spiritual path. We can frequent movies and buy books that support the growth of the human spirit, and support women producers and writers. Most important, we can "inhabit our own lives." I was at a humanistic psychology conference (where most of the attendees were women) and was both shocked and delighted when a woman, not part of the program, stepped up to the podium. She reminded us that we were attending this conference because we cared, and yet she had just witnessed a particularly careless act. Two women had rushed through a swinging door in a hurry, letting it crash into an older woman who lost her balance and fell. Since they hadn't been paying attention, the result of their carelessness had gone unnoticed. I was not alone in feeling delighted at this woman's spontaneous call to our collective conscience. Admiration for both her observation and the gutsy way she stood up to make her point resulted in a standing ovation and lots of excited corridor conversation later on. After all, what's the point of talking about kindness if we don't practice what we preach?

How often, I wonder, am I still careless in own life? When I'm preoccupied I tend to ignore sales people, picking up my purchase from them as if they were human vending machines. I'm trying to do better, complimenting cashiers on their courtesy or finding some way to acknowledge their efforts. Most times, I'm rewarded with a smile. A little energy flows between us that enlivens us both and will be passed on to other people that we interact with that day. Sometimes the cashier is too preoccupied to respond, and that's okay, too. A kind word is never wasted because it is equally uplifting to the giver as it is to the receiver. This is true not only psychologically, but also biologically. Nurse/researcher Janet Quinn of the University of Colorado, for example, did a study on a form of energy healing known as therapeutic touch (TT). The core principle of TT is the strong mental intention to transmit respect and compassion to the person being healed. The giver of TT holds a strong mental image of the receiver as whole or healthy, intending to send universal healing energy through her hands (which are held several inches away from the body of the "healee") into the energy field of the receiver. When Dr. Quinn measured the effects of TT on T-lymphocyte function, a measure of immunity, there was an improvement not only in the receiver, but also in the giver.

Sometimes seemingly small acts of kindness will touch off an explosion, a "big bang" that suddenly gives rise to a new universe of possibilities. Consider Mother Teresa, who began her mission in 1952 by picking up one dying man from a sewer in Calcutta, providing love and comfort while he passed over. In the next thirty years, she and her Sisters of Charity picked up over forty thousand more dying people. The fact that nearly half have recovered is a remarkable testimony to the healing power of love.

Psychologist David McClelland, while a professor at Harvard, did a study concerning Mother Teresa. His premise was that she modeled a psychological trait akin to unconditional love, which he called Affiliative Trust. Affiliative Trust is a willingness to open the heart, a belief that giving and receiving love is of paramount importance. After watching a documentary on the life of Mother Teresa, tests revealed not only that the viewers had more thoughts of Affiliative Trust, but also that an antibody found in saliva, called secretory immunoglobulin A (s-IgA) had risen significantly. S-IgA is the first line of defense against germs that enter through the nose and mouth and is an integral part of the body's defense against infectious disease as well as tooth decay and gingivitis. About an hour after watching the Mother Teresa film, the research subjects' s-IgA began to drop. It rose again when they were asked to close their eyes and recall a time from their own life when they were either giving or receiving love unconditionally. Affiliative Trust is a good working definition of self-in-relation, a psychospiritual state in which both people reach a higher level of health and happiness because of their interrelatedness.

Most of us, myself included, would feel completely overwhelmed at the prospect of ministering to as many people as Mother Teresa. But she writes of an attitude that completely bypasses the confusion about knowing where to start, and the numbness and paralysis that often set in when the necessary changes are so large. She writes, "I never look at the masses as my responsibility. I look at the individual. I can love only one person at a time. I can feed only one person at a time. Just one, one, one. You get closer to Christ by coming closer to each other. As Jesus said, 'Whatever you do to the least of my brethren, you do to me.' So you begin. . . . I begin. I picked up one person—maybe if I didn't pick up that one person I wouldn't have picked up forty two thousand. The whole work is only a drop in the ocean. But if I didn't put the drop in, the ocean would be one drop less. Same thing for you, same thing in your family, same thing in the church where you go. Just begin . . . one, one, one."

A FEMININE PATH TO POWER AND SOCIAL ACTION

While this is not meant to be a book on social policy, we need to consider how late midlife women can take advantage of what anthropologist Margaret Mead called their "postmenopausal zest," and what I have called the emergence of the Guardian, by being helpful to others in ways that also lead to our own happiness and longevity. The prodigious physiological changes of menopause that we have discussed in the previous two chapters have let the genie of yang, or masculine, energy, out of the bottle. Midlife testosterone levels are high in women, but in contrast to men, so are our levels of estrogen, even though they are lower than they were premenopausally. So the fear that socially active women will become a cadre of fierce, masculine warriors is not warranted by our physiology. Nor is it warranted by the psychological development of a lifetime that has been organized around the primary spiritual values of interdependency and interrelatedness.

Many women are afraid of power and success, afraid of taking leadership roles, and I believe that one of the underlying reasons for this lies in the fact that we are aware of how power has been abused through the millennia, most often by men who have been in positions of political and social ascendancy. Therefore, it is crucial to stop for a moment and consider feminine concepts of power if we are truly to pick up the mantle of the Guardian in late midlife and older adulthood.

Let's take a hypothetical look at how American history might have been different if Christopher Columbus had operated from a feminine basis of power. His long sea journey finally at an end, Columbus landed in the New World and discovered an indigenous people who lived the feminine principles of interdependence. They gave freely to one another and to Columbus and his men, honored relationship—to one another, to the earth, and to the creator, and lived the values triad of love, serenity and service. The word *Indian*, in fact, derives from the Spanish *Indios*, meaning "a people in whom God was evident." Columbus wrote back to King Ferdinand and Queen Isabella, the patrons of his journey, "So tractable, so peaceable are these people that I swear to Your Majesties there is not in the world a better nation. They love their neighbors as themselves, and their discourse is ever sweet and gentle, and accompanied with a smile."

Indian life might have exemplified a true working definition of Christianity, yet Columbus's mission, dictated by the version of power that most women fear, was to make the Indians "adopt our ways." And thus began the bloodiest, most reprehensible chapter in American history—the pillage and destruction of the people, the original Indian Nations, upon whose ashes modern America was built. Had Columbus been a woman, or a man who worked from a feminine base of power, the scenario might have switched from the conqueror trying to dominate and change the Indians, to an exchange of culture valuable to both parties. In Paul Ray's conception, the Spaniards and Indians might have been able to cocreate a mutually beneficial, respectful Integral Culture.

As the world becomes more and more of a melting pot, feminine power is increasingly important. Is the planet to become a homogeneous landscape of McDonald'ses and Walmarts, where every culture is expected to conform to the American Dream, or can we learn from other cultures, thus enriching our own?

After attending the United Nations World Conference on Women in Beijing in 1995, where over 40,000 women from 184 nations gathered to discuss the possibilities of creating a new future, Betty Friedan wrote, "The world's women now converging on Beijing suddenly loom as a great force at the very moment when deadly new games of violence and greed seem to be taking over the entire world. Are women irrelevant to those power players? They may think so; they may wish women would just stop talking about values, human rights, about the concerns of children and the environment, the old and the poor, the whole social agenda that the men now seizing power in many lands want to reverse. I know we won't stop talking."

The key to a feminine power that can inform social activism lies not in the opposition to the male power of dominion and conquest, nor in its emulation. Rather it rests on the inherent appreciation of diversity, a belief in the worth of all human beings, and the ability to honor multiple points of view that is intrinsic to the biology and psychology of women. The biological pathways of empathy that develop in early childhood, for example, are predicated on the ability to put ourselves in the place of another and understand how the other feels. When we can sense the world from another person's perspective, it makes us more tolerant. We understand that our own viewpoint is not the only one. The empathetic relationality of women also makes it more difficult to objectify another person as "the enemy," so that their rights can be discounted. When power is informed by empathy, social action can be moved to a whole new level.

In middle childhood, girls learn to reason not only with the linear logic of the mind, but also with the relational logic of the heart. Like Amy, the eleven-year-old girl whom Carol Gilligan used as an example of moral reasoning, adult women are similarly capable of appreciating the widespread ramifications of any action. Those women who are Cultural Creatives are particularly attuned to the ways our collective decisions about issues as diverse as pesticide use, educational policy, and the rising tide of crime and violence affect the overall quality of life. For example, on the plus side, pesticide use sometimes increases crop yield, making more food available. On the other hand, pesticides may pollute soil and groundwater, eventually entering the fatty tissues of animals and humans, promoting cancer growth or damaging DNA and causing mutations. Furthermore, pesticides like DDT that are banned in the United States are shipped for use on crops in Third World countries. Are the lives of their citizens less valuable than ours? Is it a reasonable trade-off to use DDT to kill mosquitoes in areas where malaria is endemic if it is cheaper than less toxic substances? Is economics the most important variable in any equation, as it has been in so many instances?

Midlife women, by sheer force of numbers and experience, are now in the position to launch a new kind of social activism informed by the intrinsic spirituality of interrelatedness, and to put their energy to work as guardians of life. Paul Ray's research on Cultural Creatives, the majority of whom are women, indicates that the urge to form a new Integral Culture based on empathetic interrelationship with diverse people and the environment is widespread, involving nearly one quarter of all Americans. But in order to bring a new social order of Integral Culture into being, we need to reflect continually on what it is to be truly in relation, truly in a spirit of service. Otherwise it is easy to slip into the old model of having power over another person, institution, or culture because we think our way is better.

Physician Rachel Naomi Remen, a midlife woman who is medical director of the Commonweal Cancer Help Program in Bolinas, California, and author of *Kitchen Table Wisdom*, writes about the difference between service as a form of connection with life, and service that is a veiled form of judgment, a statement that someone is broken and needs fixing. "In fixing there is an inequality of expertise that can easily become a moral distance. We cannot serve at a distance. We can only serve that to which we are profoundly connected, that which we are willing to touch. This is Mother Teresa's basic message. We serve life not because it is broken but because it is holy."

THE HEART OF A WOMAN: A ROLE MODEL FOR SPIRIT IN ACTION

An old Cheyenne proverb states that "A nation is not conquered until the hearts of its women are on the ground. Then it is done, no matter how brave its warriors or how strong their weapons." In this section I want to feature the work of one woman who exemplifies what any of us can do when social service is driven by the feminine values of interrelatedness and respect. Her name is Robin Casarjian, a midlife woman from Boston, Massachusetts. The issue she has chosen to bring her heart to is reform of the criminal justice system.

Robin didn't set out to become a prison reformer, but simply responded in a heartfelt way to needs as they appeared in her life. While teaching stress management at the Harvard Community Health Plan in the 1980s, Robin became increasingly convinced that lack of forgiveness was a frequently overlooked source of stress for many people. She became well known for her interest in the topic and was asked to give a talk on forgiveness at MCI Gardner, a medium-security prison in Massachusetts housing seven hundred men. Incredibly, one hundred twenty men showed up for the talk and listened with rapt attention for two hours. There was a hunger for knowledge, a hunger for healing. So Robin responded to the need by volunteering to present a fifteen-session course on forgiveness and emotional healing at the prison.

Over the next several years, she presented many such sessions both in men's and women's prisons, learning some astonishing facts about crime and punishment in the process. The facts you are about to read come from a newsletter of the Lionheart Foundation, a nonprofit project dedicated to turning prisons into houses of healing that Robin founded in 1992. The punishment industry (prisons and juvenile detention centers) is currently the fastest-growing sector of the economy. One and a half million Americans are now behind bars, a fivefold increase since 1970, with a weekly net increase of two thousand prisoners. It would require building four new prisons a week to accommodate this explosive growth. One study revealed that if the prison population continues to grow at its current rate, more than half the country will be in jail by the middle of the next century. That, naturally, would bankrupt the government. The sad fact is that nearly one in three black males in their twenties are under the control of the criminal justice system (in jail, on parole, on probation); one in eight young Hispanic males; one in fifteen young white males. Three quarters of all prisoners in New York State (nearly seventy thousand people) come from seven communities in New York City, which are typical blighted inner-city neighborhoods. The poverty, disease, poor infant health, and rampant unemployment there are a recipe for despondency, hopelessness, and crime. More than 50 percent of the boys in these neighborhoods are high school dropouts, and there is a 60 percent unemployment rate for black males.

But there are some rays of hope. Inmates who enter drug- and alcohol-recovery programs, for example, are only half as likely to go back to jail as those who do not. A study done in California found that every dollar spent on such programs saved seven dollars in future costs. Likewise, inmates who finish college have an extremely low recidivism rate—only 7 percent—but the Pell Grants for college tuition that gave so many prisoners hope have been cut because of politicians who refuse to "coddle" criminals. Many people want retribution, and they consider educational, psychological, and spiritual programs a form of "going soft" on offenders. Compassionate, effective rehabilitation, however, is not coddling. It calls offenders to take responsibility for their actions, while healing the underlying problems in empathetic relationality that allow them to victimize others because they are unable to put themselves in another person's place. Whenever the ability to understand another's rights or feelings is lacking, it becomes easy to see them as something less than we are and to take advantage of them emotionally, politically, criminally, or militarily.

Robin's vision is that prisons should be houses of healing, places where people can become emotionally literate, learn to forgive themselves and others, and break out of the cycle of abuse and hopelessness. She routinely works with murderers, burglars, sex offenders, and drug traffickers, assuring us with the light of a proud parent in her eyes that given meaningful guidance and support, many can heal and become loving, caring, human beings. Robin's gift is that she sees their lights, not their lampshades (a phrase coined by psychiatrist Jerry Jampolsky), providing the sacred space of respect and encouragement in which healing and transformation can occur.

In 1992 Robin's magnificent book called *Forgiveness: A Bold Choice for a Peaceful Heart* was published. When it came time to write a second book, she decided to write it especially and exclusively for prisoners. This is the kind of book for which there are no advances, no publishers clamoring at your door, no accolades, and no money to be made. In fact, in order to write, publish, and distribute the book, which is entitled *Houses of Healing: A Prisoner's Guide to Inner Power and Freedom*, Robin founded the nonprofit Lionheart Foundation. By early 1996 she had accomplished most of the first phase of its mission. Multiple copies of the book had been distributed to all federal prisons, and state prisons in most states. Robin also published a workbook for prison staff who wish to implement the program, and after these materials are in all the nation's prisons the second phase of the work will begin—a Spanish-language edition, and audiotapes for those who are illiterate. Letters pour in daily from grateful inmates who have checked the book out of their prison libraries. In some institutions there is thankfully, but unfortunately, a long waiting list to read it. And although many prisoners have requested personal copies of *Houses of Healing*, more money needs to be raised to provide individual copies as well as completing distribution to prison libraries and translating the book into Spanish and making audiotape versions. If you'd like to make a donation, please send it to the Lionheart Foundation, Box 194, Back Bay, Boston, MA 02117.

THE GIFTS OF ALTRUISM AND SERVICE

Through the years I've met so many women who have an eagerness to help, but don't know what they can do. Robin's advice is this. "If you don't have a strong inner guidance, something you might do if you want to make a difference is to ask yourself, 'Who is it I feel most drawn to serve? Is it children, the elderly, the homeless?' Once that question is answered, look at what the options are—volunteering at a school, being a Big Sister, visiting the elderly, cleaning the neighborhood, working "behind the scenes" for an organization, doing child care for a single parent, sharing time with your own aging parent. The opportunities to serve are all around us constantly. Every interaction is an opportunity to serve, to share love and goodwill."

When we share that love and goodwill, giving is not a one-way street. There is an old adage that whatever we give away comes back to us. We receive what we give. In terms of health, the gifts of giving result in a stronger immune system, fewer illnesses, and a longer life. As a health strategy alone, service makes sense. From a psychological perspective, compassionate, caring service helps to alleviate depression. When we are in relation to the person we are helping we feel renewed, more creative, and more peaceful. The self-esteem generated by service keeps hopelessness from taking root. From a spiritual perspective, service is a good working definition of spirituality in action. The Jewish faith is firmly based in the practice of mitzvot, acts of kindness, compassion, and service to others. These are considered the highest form of prayer. Jesus, who was a first-century rabbi, carried these strong teachings on service into what later became Christianity. The heart of Buddhism is likewise based on altruistic service with the understanding that since all things are interdependent, what we do for anyone else, we also do for ourselves. Without others, we wouldn't have the opportunity to become better human beings.

When we come into our fullness as Guardians of life, bearing the standards of a new Integral Culture based on the feminine values triad of love, serenity, and service, we simultaneously increase our own happiness, health, and longevity. Every act of kindness and compassion toward others gets multiplied when they, in turn, pass it on. One by one the world becomes a better place. Service is indeed the gift that keeps on giving.

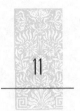

11

AGES 63–70: WISDOM'S DAUGHTERS

CREATING A NEW INTEGRAL CULTURE

Julia was sound asleep, wrapped in the shifting images of a strangely vivid dream. Her mother, Sylvia, was a young woman of about thirty-five, dressed in Victorian garb—a white bustled dress and wide-brimmed hat with trailing ribbons. Standing on the deck of an ocean liner, she shaded herself from the bright sun with a lace-trimmed parasol, the sky above her an unearthly shade of azure blue that blended into the surface of a glassy ocean. Sylvia was waving a gay good-bye to Julia, who in the dream was her actual age, sixty-four, although she felt as forlorn as a child. Looking up at the ship from the dock below, Julia was begging her mother not to go on the trip. Tears were streaming down her face. But Sylvia seemed unconcerned. "Be happy for me," she shouted, "I'm going home to John and I've missed him so much."

Julia tried to reason with her mother. "But Daddy's dead and you live in Brookline. You can't go away. You'll get lost. You'll get lost," she shouted. But her mother's laughter carried on the wind. "No, Julia, I'm not going to get lost, I'm finding myself. I'm going home. You'll be all right. Everything is all right. I've waited so long for my freedom. Please be happy for me." The scene shifted and Julia found herself in her mother's arms. "I love you, Caterpillar," Sylvia whispered into Julia's hair as she addressed her daughter by a childhood nickname, "and I'll always be with you, no matter where you are."

Suddenly Julia found herself back on the dock and the great steamship began to pull away, blasts of its horn signaling the departure, and rousing Julia from the dream world as the sound mutated into the insistent ringing of her bedside telephone. It was a call from the hospital, alerting Julia that her ninety-year-old mother had called 911 when she awakened with chest pains at about 5 A.M. She had been admitted to the coronary intensive care unit and was asking for her daughter.

Julia was dressed and out the door in five minutes, and at the hospital half an hour later. All the while she prayed for her mother to hang on until she got there, so that they could say good-bye, or at least so that she could say good-bye. Julia felt with a poignant certainty that her mother had already said good-bye in her dream, and was ready to leave this life. When Julia got to the hospital, she was allowed only ten minutes with Sylvia, a rule that was supposed to let the patients in the cardiac intensive care unit rest, and also spare the nursing staff some of the congestion that visitors could create.

Sylvia was weak and pale, but quite coherent. Julia told her mother about the dream, crying when she reached the part about Sylvia's pledge always to be there for her, and cradling her mother's thin hand, with its fine parchmentlike skin, next to her heart. Looking deeply into her mother's eyes Julia told her how much she would miss her, but that she understood that it was time for her mother to go now. Sylvia squeezed her daughter's hand, and said, "I'm almost ready, but there are a few more good-byes I'd like to say." She paused and closed her eyes to rest for a moment. "I've had the nurse call your brother, Alex, and he's flying up from Florida. God willing he'll be here this afternoon. I'm only sorry there's not enough time for Amanda and Benjamin to come."

Julia started to protest, "But, Mom, there is time, I'll call them right now. They can arrange to be here by tomorrow or even tonight." Sylvia looked so peaceful against her pillows, even with the IV fluids flowing into her veins and the constant beep of the cardiac monitors resounding throughout the unit. She squeezed Julia's hand again. "Tomorrow's probably too late, my love. I can hang on till Alex comes, but after that, I don't know. Whenever I close my eyes," she continued dreamily, "I see a kind of filmy light, a warm light, and a kind of deep azure blue sky. I see John waiting for me, and my parents," Sylvia paused as if actually seeing the scene she was narrating to Julia. "I'm ready to go to them, darling. I feel half there already. . . . I just had to see you and Alex one last time."

Their ten minutes were quickly over and Julia bent down to kiss her mother, then left to start the process of having Sylvia moved out of the intensive care unit to a regular private room where she could die surrounded by family and friends, with unlimited visiting hours. Sylvia left her body peacefully at ten A.M. the following morning with both her children, and her son-in-law, Roger, by her side. As Julia sat with her mother for the twenty-four hours it took for Sylvia to say her goodbyes and transit from this world to the next, she began to think of the generations of her family like waves, cresting and rolling toward shore. Sylvia's wave had just arrived on land, delivering her home. Her own wave, and that of her husband, were cresting now in their elder years, and would be the next wave to break on the shore. Behind them were the waves of their children and grandchildren, four generations in all. She and Roger had lived through three quarters of the wheel of life and were now in its final quadrant, the wisdom years.

Julia was fortunate in having a mother who was a model of vitality and continued growth in the last quarter of her life. Sylvia lived for ninety years in good health, due at least in part to the fact that she had always taken good care of herself, stayed involved with people, and offered her services whenever she could. A lifetime of intellectual pursuit kept her mind growing. She volunteered at a homeless shelter every Sunday and led book-discussion groups at the senior apartment complex where she had lived independently until the time of her death. Because she was respected as an elder, and had the opportunity to share the wisdom of a lifetime with family and friends, Sylvia also remained strong emotionally. One of the family jokes revolved around Sylvia's habit of answering the telephone with a line once spoken by Lucy in a Peanuts comic strip, "The psychiatrist is in now, please deposit five cents."

The stereotype of aging as a progressive loss of function is generally true only for people who stop functioning. The adage "Use it or lose it" is a powerful truth for the last quarter of life. In this and the other two chapters on the elder years there will be relatively little biology to consider because, at least in our current scientific understanding, physical development is essentially complete, although the brain continues to myelinate new pathways in response to intellectual stimulation until the very moment of our death. The ideal in a woman's elder years is to preserve the biological function that she has matured into at menopause, and to continue her psychological and spiritual development as a truthteller who continually calls both people and institutions to their highest potential.

In many ways, the life cycle is like a spiral on which we revisit earlier epochs from a higher perspective. The young girl in the first quarter of life has not yet donned the masks of social acceptability that act as a censor for what she says. She calls things as she sees them, and is frequently embarrassingly honest. We begin to lose our voice in adolescence as the constraints of culture and the dictum "Be nice, hide your feelings" puts a lid on sharing our perceptions and intuitions. Throughout our early and middle adulthood we regain our voices, and by the last quarter of life most of us are once again as outspoken as we were as girls. If we have used our lives wisely, healed old wounds, and continued developing empathy, the truth we speak will be wise and compassionate. If we have not, it may be bitter and destructive. Having finally surmounted the inhibitory injunction "If I say that, what will other people think of me?" many older women are blunt in their honesty.

My mother, Lillian, was a case in point. I'd phone her up, and after the small talk was over, she'd often be quick to point out certain essential truths about the way I was conducting my life at the time. A typical conversation went something like this: "You let your boss walk all over you. Who the hell does he think he is anyway, Simon Legree? He runs an intellectual sweat shop over there. You're working sixty hours a week, for heaven's sake. And what do you get paid? Peanuts. Crabs in ice water. You're worth a lot more. What's wrong with you, anyway. Why don't you stick up for yourself, Joani? You're acting like a dope. Think about it. You don't have enough time for Justin and Andrei.

Don't you think they're paying a price because you won't speak up? You don't have any time for yourself, either. When's the last time you took a vacation or even went shopping to buy a new dress? Sometimes you look like a poster child for Goodwill Thrift Shops. Give me that blankety-blank's phone number (my mother swore a lot more as she aged) and I'll set him straight. He'll never know what hit him."

She was right. Unfortunately, tact was not her long suit and she often spoke the truth in a way that was difficult for me to hear. Her internal censor seemed to have gone off the job sometime in her sixties and she had an uncanny way of getting to the heart of matters. She considered herself somewhat of an oracle, in fact, and would only half-jokingly end her truth-telling sessions by deepening her already husky voice and proclaiming with great ceremony, "I have spoken."

A ROLE MODEL FOR ENTERING THE WISDOM YEARS

My mother was a wise woman, but as you may appreciate, not always a gentle one. Rather than making a new life for herself when my father died while they were both in their midsixties, she isolated herself, becoming progressively more bitter about life. Rather than lifting herself out of depression by reaching out to others, she turned inward to a solitary world of books and television game shows. What she said was on target, but the way that she said it often hindered other people from listening wholeheartedly.

I feel fortunate in having another elder role model who combines the ability to tell the truth with the relational skills needed in order to be heard. I had the good fortune to meet Celia Thaxter Hubbard when she was sixty-eight years old. The great-granddaughter of New England Transcendentalist poet Celia Thaxter, her namesake, Celia the younger is a renowned photographer and artist. Armed with a selection of cameras, from a fancy Nikon to a little Kodak 110 point and shoot, Celia has helped open my eyes to the beauty all around us. We've combed the beaches of Cape Cod looking for the heart-shaped stones, bits of glass, seaweed and shells that Celia believes God leaves as evidence that we are loved. Photos of hearts left when the cat's milk dries in the bowl, or a cigarette pack is run over by a car, litter her worktable, waiting to be chosen for the book she is working on, *Cosmic Valentines.*

Celia's halo of gray hair and charming wrinkles, surrounding eyes full of love, mischief, and curiosity, give her the look of a wise child. She dresses with flair, often layering colorful jackets and ethnic jewelry over fleece pants and shirts, to keep out the drafts of the renovated barn she inhabits on a historic street in Cambridge, Massachusetts. At seventy-five, she can often be seen out walking her long-haired Corgie, Sophie, and visiting companionably with friends and neighbors. Celia is ever ready with a kind word or a helping hand. She counsels many people informally through what she jokingly refers to as her "public practice."

Through the years of our friendship, Celia's lively interest in religion and spirituality has been a continuing education for me as is the stream of book recommendations, articles, and videos she is constantly bringing to my attention. Celia is ever in the process of discovery, full of news flashes about this world and the world to come. The latest advances in health care, alternative medicine, psychology, and theology are always at hand through Celia's penchant for informing herself and others. And without doubt, Celia is simply the cutest human being I've ever met. She doesn't try to look young. Why should she? She is ageless as only the discoverers amongst us can remain.

Before I met Celia, I feared growing old because I had no positive role models for the process. I didn't want to become sedentary and uninterested in life as had my mother, who just let herself go physically, socially, and intellectually after my father's death. Neither did I want to become the kind of brittle, skinny, overly madeup older woman who resembles what a friend's mother calls a "bag of antlers," and tries foolishly and fruitlessly to look the way she did at forty. But through Celia's example, I've realized that old is an attitude rather than an age.

There is a term called the "young-old" for people like Celia, demonstrating that the previous distinctions between life stages are blurring. The young-old may be sixty-five or ninety—vital, active in life, interested in the problems of society, and in no way representative of the decrepit, marginalized, senile caricature that has become ensconced in the mass mind. A woman's latter years of discovery, wisdom, and vision have been portrayed as a period of progressive degeneration, both physical and mental. And nothing could be further from the truth.

Women have been fed a bill of goods about menstruation, childbirth, menopause, and powerlessness that we are slowly overcoming. Aging is the final frontier of our freedom, the final attitude that needs to be put right. And just as the growing numbers of midlife women are rising up and claiming their power, so are the elders whose numbers are swelling in truly historic proportions.

THE AGING MAJORITY

Once again, women who are entering the wise years are on the leading edge of a revolution. We are a country in which the fastest-growing segment of the population is over sixty-five. Two trends account for this. The first is that in less than one hundred years the average age of death for women has gone from forty-seven to seventy-five, largely due to the control of infectious disease, and reductions in infant and maternal mortality. The second is the declining birthrate. In fact, the number of Americans over sixty-five has nearly tripled between 1950 and 1992, representing over 32 million people—which, for purposes of comparison, is more than the entire population of Canada—and about one eighth the population of the United States. Furthermore, the great majority of those over sixty-five are women, who outnumber men 19 to 13 million. By the year 2010 the leading edge of baby boomers—now in midlife—will start to retire, and by 2035, close to one in four Americans will be sixty-five or over.

This graying of the population will be offset by a reduction in the numbers of the young. Researchers Alan Pfifer and Lydia Brontë cite statistics that confirm a significant drop in reproductive rate, bottoming out in the mid-1970s—a "baby bust" following the baby boom. They write, "In an aging society, it is inevitable that there will be fewer households with children. Today, fewer than 38 percent of households nationwide contain anyone under eighteen years of age, compared with nearly 50 percent in 1960." This trend, of course, applies only to Western industrialized countries. In the Third World, populations still are growing exponentially, creating greater and greater poverty, which in turn leads to increased pollution and environmental devastation.

KEEPERS OF THE FLAME

For the first time in American history, the flame is being passed from the youth to the elders. Until recently, we were a young country not only in terms of our scant two hundred-year history, but in terms of the age of our citizens. In 1800, half the population was under the age of sixteen, and very few lived past sixty. The country was settled, and the West won (or lost, depending on whether you adopt a cowboy or an Indian point of view) by the young. Eliza Pinckney was seventeen when she took over managing the family's five thousand-acre North Carolina plantation in 1740, a common situation for frontier women in a sparsely populated land where men were often called away to war. George Washington was a colonel, and commander-in-chief of the Virginia Militia, at just twenty-three.

Times have changed dramatically and the population is no longer young, but views on aging have not kept pace, especially for women. Aging men often retain an aura of power, and politicians especially seem exempt from the myth that we lose creativity and worth at the magical age of sixty-five, when we are expected to retire. Like the ancient Chinese, and the French, English, and eighteenth-century Americans who once wore powdered wigs to simulate age, contemporary Americans believe that men (at least those in power) continue to grow in wisdom throughout the life span. While John F. Kennedy and Bill Clinton were midlife presidents, Ronald Reagan was elected to his first term at seventy, and his successor, George Bush, was sixty-five when he took over the Oval Office.

But for women, aging is not generally viewed as a time of wisdom and power. It is more akin to a booby prize. Getting old may be better than dying young, but it is not something that most of us have been raised to look forward to. Those of us who came of age in the 1960s, when the war cry was "Don't trust anyone over thirty" are ill prepared for our sixties unless we've been doing some more recent radical thinking. The old ways of our society—materialism, militarism, and lack of equal rights for women and people of color—were rejected as immoral and untenable by the sixties generation. But we were young and destined to come into wisdom gradually, as nature intended. We did not lose the dream of peace and freedom, as some believe, we have just been maturing into it.

As the "flower children" married, found careers, and bore children, most of us were assimilated into the very system that we had rebelled against, gleaning a firsthand knowledge of its workings that cannot be had in youth. Now an entire generation of midlifers and sixty-somethings are reawakening to the old vision. What we didn't realize in the youthful idealism that trusted no one over thirty is that we were rebelling against an old system, not old people. And now that we ourselves are aging, those of us who have held the vision of cooperation, compassion, equality, and peace finally have the experience and power to bring it to fruition. We even have a new name, the Cultural Creatives, and a new mission, the founding of an Integral Culture based on the feminine values of interdependence and relationality. But in order to claim that power we must first confront the prejudices against aging.

THE AGING MYSTIQUE

Betty Friedan, who opened a new world to women in 1963 when *The Feminine Mystique* was published, has written an equally illuminating book on aging. In *The Fountain of Age* she writes, "I have discovered that there is a crucial difference between society's image of old people and 'us' as we know and feel ourselves to be." So pervasive is our fear of age, argues Friedan, that we have neatly edited it out of our lives. She cites numerous examples of age discrimination, some of which are listed below, including one study of prime-time network television that monitored TV dramas for a week. Out of 464 character portrayals, only seven (1.5 percent) looked to be sixty-five or older. In a similar vein, out of 290 faces in Vogue, only one woman was clearly over sixty, and that in a little inset called "me and granny." (There were, however, four "power shots" of older men.) Similarly, out of 265 articles on aging in a major midwestern newspaper, none featured elders in a positive light. Every article focused on problems. Friedan concluded that the aging mystique was even more deadly than the feminine mystique she called to our attention in the 1960s.

Challenging the feminine mystique, which cast women as appendages and helpmates of men, who had the real power, was a necessary step in the birth of the new wave of Cultural Creatives (CCs) who are at the leading edge of social reform. According to sociologist Paul Ray, CCs began to solidify into a social, cultural worldview in the 1970s, and there is no question that the women's movement was an important impetus in informing and disseminating the values that characterize CCs, including an interest in women's issues, relationships, psychology, spirituality, alternative health care, and a strong stance for the protection of children, the environment, and the Third World.

CCs already represent 24 percent of all Americans. The growth of this new cultural worldview, which got an important boost from challenging the feminine mystique, will get a second major boost from challenging the aging mystique. When both women and men are liberated from the myth that elders are useless, the enormous pool of talent latent in the growing ranks of older Americans can be mobilized to bring forth the Integral Culture that Paul Ray sees looming on the horizon. If elders use their retirement years to become involved in social and political action, not only will their own health and longevity benefit, but they can potentially turn the cultural tide from the prevalent values of Modernism to a Transmodern, relational way of looking at the world. Ray postulates that our Modernist institutions of work, education, and business will endure, but in new forms based on more feminine values. He writes, "The possibility of a new culture centers on reintegration of what has been fragmented by Modernism: self-integration and authenticity; integration with community and connection with others around the globe, not just at home; connection with nature and learning to integrate ecology and economy; and a synthesis of diverse views and traditions, including philosophies of East and West. Thus, *Integral* Culture."

The debunking of the aging mystique and the rise of Integral Culture will, I believe, go hand in hand, creating an exciting new mission for aging Americans, and reframing the meaning of retirement. If we retired from our conventional work so that we could dedicate ourselves to a working for a new cultural ideal, aging would become the most vital time of life, a time to rebirth the world culture. Janet Sainer, who retired from her position as commissioner of the New York Department of Aging at the age of seventy to become a consultant to both the governments of the United States and Israel, speaks of the dangers of what she calls the "retirement mystique." The idea that we are used up at sixty-five, she believes, is patently ridiculous. Why waste the experience of a lifetime, which is so sorely needed by business, industry, education, social services, and the government? Sainer blames discrimination against the aging on two sources: the media and gerontology researchers. The former thrives on hard-luck stories and fear mongering. The latter focus their research on pathology rather than potential. By focusing on the sick minority, the mere 5 percent of Americans over sixty-five who are in nursing homes, they have ignored the vital majority (and remember that most of these are women) and the contributions they can make not only in their sixties, but into their eighties and beyond.

CULTURAL DIFFERENCES: WISDOM'S DAUGHTERS OR SOCIETY'S LEFTOVERS?

Aging white women have precious few role models to look to because the aging mystique has disempowered so many of our elders. Black, Hispanic, and Native American cultures, in contrast, venerate older women. These cultures view women elders as becoming more wise and beautiful than they were before, rather than fading into something physically, emotionally, and spiritually less than they were in their youth. Wise elders are a tremendous source of knowledge, having lived long enough to understand the delicate, and sometimes invisible, web of interconnections that link our every action to a network of tangible and intangible results.

Betty Laverdure is an Ojibwa of the Bear Clan, a tribal judge and legislator, who has been recognized as an elder since the age of forty-five, when she was given the honorable title Grandmother. She says, "Grandmother, that wonderful name, has always meant teacher in all of our society. That's a good distinction and I'm proud of it." In describing her own grandmother, a revered medicine woman, she says, "Her name meant like you throw a rock in the water and the ripples are so far-reaching. As I've aged, I've come to view a successful woman in just this way, as a person whose thoughts, words and actions send out far-reaching ripples that touch others in positive ways."

In Ojibwa and many other Native American cultures, women are revered because they are thought to be in especially close connection to the Great Mystery. Traditional Native women are indeed exquisitely attuned to the natural world, and to the interconnectedness of the seasons, the plants, the festivals, the holy days, the harvest. They are prone to the kind of prescient dreams and intuitions that Julia had of her mother's impending death. In past times, all major decisions were made in consultation with women elders whose feminine apprehension of the interconnectedness of various facets of life allowed them to see how any "stone thrown into the water" would affect the tribe and the earth seven generations into the future. If the result of any action would not be beneficial in the future, it was vetoed. Can you imagine how different our world might be if the compassionate, empathetic, interdependent, intuitive wisdom of the feminine—which is potentially present both in men and in women—was the final arbiter of affairs of state?

THE ORACLE: RECLAIMING THE FEMININE WISDOM OF INTERDEPENDENCE

An oracle is a truth teller, and the truth is not always pleasant for those bent on preserving the status quo. If, like Native Americans, women had the power to veto war, our oracle would be a deathblow to the enormous military-industrial complex on which the United States', and indeed the world's, economy hinges. Many truths are painfully evident, like the fact that 80 percent of all cancers are related to environmental pollution. Furthermore, common pollutants like lead, which is found in paint and in the soil where it is deposited through automobile exhaust, causes mental retardation in children. Both lead and polychorinated biphenyls (PCBs), which are by-products of the manufacture of electrical components and enter the food chain through the soil and water, have been linked to violent behavior in children.

In 1996, *Time, Newsweek,* the major newspaper chains, and a spate of books called public attention to the fact that pesticides based on a class of chlorine containing molecules called organochlorines have estrogenlike activity. These molecules are called *xenoestrogens* (from *xeno*, meaning "foreign") because they come from outside the body. They then bind to receptor sites for estradiol in the body, mimicking its biological action. Although further research is needed, preliminary studies link xenoestrogens to the development of prostate cancer in men, and breast and ovarian cancer in women. Furthermore, xenoestrogens may affect the gonads of developing fetuses, leading to reduced fertility. When I attempted to do a literature search on the behavioral effects of PCBs by accessing the National Library of Medicine on my computer, I was shocked to find that several thousand articles were listed.

Biologist Rachel Carson was an oracle when *Silent Spring*, the first popular book on pesticides, was published in 1962 when she was in her sixties. She had meticulously researched the environmental effects of DDT and other pesticides that she felt were being used indiscriminately without regard for how they affected the delicate balance of nature. She predicted that the poisoning of the air, water, and earth by these chemicals would eventually lead to the death of most insects, birds, and small animals, until one day we would have a silent spring. Her thesis was attacked by chemical companies who tried hard to silence her. But her voice prevailed. President John F. Kennedy appointed a special scientific advisory committee to investigate pesticides.

The use of DDT was eventually banned in this country, but unfortunately it is still shipped out for use in Third World countries and we eventually get it back on produce that is shipped to us. Like most pesticides, DDT is fat soluble, otherwise it would wash off crops during rainstorms or irrigation. Once these pesticides enter body fat, their half-life (the time it takes for half the amount to disappear from the body) can be many years. When mothers breast-feed, however, body fat is mobilized and pesticides and other pollutants are released into breast milk. In 1976, while I was lecturing on the structure and function of the breast at Tufts Medical School, I came across a chilling statistic. Nearly half of all lactating women who had been tested had levels of PCBs in their breast milk higher than the government deemed safe. I'm not suggesting that formulas are any better, since pollutants accumulate in cow's milk just as they do in human milk, and there are many important reasons why breast-feeding is best for infants. I am suggesting that the pollution of mother's milk—the most literal, as well as highly symbolic, giver of life—transforms it instead into the bearer of death. Are the PCBs in mother's milk causing cancer or violent behavior in their children? Will formula produced from the milk of cows reared on organically grown produce eventually be the only safe option for our babies? What more powerful impetus could we have to clean up our air, soil and water that we might preserve the health and quality of life for our children and our children's children.

When the feminine voice has opposed expansionism in Western culture, it has almost always been silenced. Wise women elders like Betty Friedan, theologist/environmentalist Rosemary Radford Ruether, and children's advocate Marion Wright Edelman are now speaking out in increasing numbers. Because of the vast increase in our numbers, and the fact that we outnumber men two to one, women elders have an unprecedented opportunity to speak out against pollution and oppose chemical companies who would silence us, to speak out against domestic violence and push through legislation that would require abusive men to enter rehabilitation programs, to speak out against cuts in the education and child-services sectors that would deprive our children of the opportunity to develop into morally, intellectually, and emotionally competent adults.

Rosemary Radford Ruether, a professor of theology at Garrett-Evangelical Theological Seminary in Evanston, Illinois, is a wise woman elder and spiritually centered social activist. She is the leader of a movement based on the idea that spirituality and the preservation of the earth are interrelated concepts. Ruether calls for a new awareness that the earth itself is a living entity, a belief that Native American and other indigenous cultures have always had. Two biologists, James Lovelock and Lynn Margulis, have dubbed the living earth Gaia, the ancient Greek word for "earth goddess."

In her magnificent book, *Gaia and God*, Ruether speaks of transforming the old system of exploiting the earth for the natural resources to fuel war and industrial expansion into a new system based on the guardianship of a living, evolving planet. Speaking of our current military system she writes, "It is their system of power that is the true 'enemy of humanity' and of the earth. But the dismantling of this system of destructive power demands real 'conversion,' a *metanoia*, or change of heart and consciousness. This change of consciousness is one that recognizes that real 'security' lies, not in the dominating power and the impossible quest for total invulnerability, but rather in the acceptance of vulnerability, limits, and interdependency with others, with other humans and with the earth." Grandmothers of wisdom, like Rosemary Radford Ruether, are issuing a call for a societal change of heart, a call that is being heeded by the growing number of Cultural Creatives.

THE ORACULAR BIOLOGY OF WOMEN'S WISDOM

Another woman elder, Marian Diamond, has done some fascinating research that indicates that the female brain continues to evolve throughout the life cycle in ways that support interdependent, oracular thinking. Diamond is a Berkeley neuroscientist, now in her seventies, who uses her own prodigious and continuously growing mental capacities to study how stimulation and aging affect neural circuitry. Her office is filled with interesting artifacts, among them pieces of Albert Einstein's brain, which she keeps in a mayonnaise jar. Diamond and her colleagues studied the effect of enriched environments (lots of playthings and mazes that were changed at frequent intervals) on the development of rats' brains. Enriched young rats, compared to those living in standard wire cages, grew larger brains. But enriched older rats also showed brain growth at a time when brain size normally diminishes. Diamond interprets her results as evidence that our brains maintain plasticity—the ability to make new functional connections—into old age.

Brain morphology, or basic structure, also changes with age in a way that may be related to the development of oracular wisdom. Diamond found that patterns of laterality (the relative thickness of the right versus the left cerebral hemispheres) change with aging. In the female (rats at least), certain parts of the right hemisphere thicken substantially. These changes are affected by factors such as stress and sex hormones, and she hypothesizes that they should also relate to changes in behavior. While cautioning that we don't yet understand the behavioral changes that this reversal of laterality might support, she speculates that in a rat's younger years a larger left cortex would be advantageous because it would lead to increased vocalization (language is a left-hemispheric function), which a female needs both for her own protection and in order to call her young and ensure their well-being. In our older years, a larger right cortex might be advantageous because of the increase in intuitive, imaginative, interdependent thinking it would theoretically support.

THE GIFTS OF THE WISDOM YEARS

When writer/photographer Steve Wall was visiting Indian reservations to interview Native American women elders, an old woman approached him, saying that word had gotten around about his project. Without identifying herself, this mysterious Grandmother announced, "There are forces at work most of us do not want to acknowledge. Only now do we understand enough to be given these things. I come to you on the feminine side, because *this is the time of the woman*, time of the feminine. We have our prophecies, and these things must come out. . . . Spiritual communications come through the feminine side. Oh, there is nothing wrong with the masculine. Action is masculine. Producing is masculine, but there must be balance."

For many years it has been the time of the masculine, and our society has profited in many ways through the male principles of activity and production. It is time now, however, for the pendulum to swing back toward the feminine so that a physically healthy earth and an emotionally healthy world population can be preserved and encouraged. By the time we have reached our midsixties, many of us find ourselves relatively free from the concerns of our younger years—taking care of children or earning a living. If we use these freedom years productively, to help create a shift into an Integral Culture that values nature as well as technology, that honors diversity and the opportunity that different cultures have to learn from one another, we will not only help to preserve our health and foster longevity, but we will also usher a new worldview into being.

By keeping active and involved in the world and by using our voices, we can truly become grandmothers of vision. And with nature's simple elegance, the more we use our wisdom, the more the neural circuitry that supports it will continue to develop. Perhaps the next generation will look back on the elders of the late twentieth century as the foremothers of a new millennium in which the spirit of relationality restored balance to a troubled world.

AGES 70–77:
THE GIFTS OF CHANGE

RESILIENCY, LOSS, AND GROWTH

At seventy-three, Julia is the director of an eldering project on the Roxbury-Jamaica Plain border on the outskirts of Boston's Harvard Medical Area. The project took three years to develop and implement, and has received national reknown as a model of a multiracial, multiethnic center that focuses not only on how elders can best be served by the community, but how the community can be served and enriched by its elders.

The planning years were a difficult balancing act between Julia's professional and personal lives. She had been working part-time for nearly twenty years, and assuming the directorship of the eldering project required her to make close to a full-time work commitment in her late sixties, coincident with Roger's being diagnosed with chronic lymphocytic leukemia just before his eighty-first birthday. They had both carefully considered the offer for Julia to spearhead the project, understanding that it would require a commitment that would reduce the amount of time they had to spend together, time that was clearly limited by Roger's health.

When Julia accepted the position, it was on her terms, with the understanding that she could take one month of unpaid vacation every three months. During those times she and Roger had traveled back to Bangladesh and India, spent time in a rented oceanfront cottage on Martha's Vineyard, and compiled a book about their family's roots. They had traveled both to England and Italy to trace the family tree through several generations so that their two children and five grandchildren, who ranged in age from four to thirteen when Roger's leukemia was diagnosed, could understand their heritage. They even discovered that Roger's great-grandfather was half Seminole Indian, and included legends and stories from the Seminole tradition in their "Family History Book."

The book grew, over two years' time, to have its own legendary importance for the family. Amanda and Benjamin became involved in the research as did their spouses, who began to trace their own family tree so that the children could understand their complete genealogy. Poetry, history, literature, mythology, and folktales from each ancestral country enriched the book, as did stories and photos from Roger and Julia's long marriage.

Since chronic lymphocytic leukemia tends to progress very slowly, Roger stayed relatively healthy and energetic up until the last six months of his life. This last period was the most difficult time for Julia, both because the nearness of Roger's death became more real each day, and also because the eldering project had just opened and required more time than it had in the planning phase. Every hour that Roger and Julia spent together seemed like a gift, and it became progressively more difficult for her to leave their home in the mornings to go to work. As Roger grew weaker, he and Julia made plans for what they called a "loving, conscious death." If possible, Roger wanted to die at home rather than in the hospital. And if he happened to be hospitalized when it was clear that his life was near the end, he did not want any heroic measures to be taken to prolong his life. He signed a do-not-resuscitate (DNR) order as his mother-in-law, Sylvia, had done, and also considered the possibility that he might choose to forgo food and water when death seemed imminent. With his disease, however, the imminence of death could be forestalled periodically by blood transfusions as an outpatient.

When he began to become seriously anemic within a week of his last transfusion, Roger let Julia know that he was ready to die, and did not want any further treatment. She took a leave of absence from work and with daily help from the hospice nurse who had already been visiting Roger weekly, transformed their bedroom into what Roger jokingly called "the birthing suite," where he was getting ready, very seriously, to give birth to his soul. On the morning when he did so, he was surrounded by loved ones. Julia, Amanda, Benjamin, and several of his friends were there when he slipped into a final, peaceful sleep.

Loss, Grief, and Resiliency

Women in their late sixties and seventies are at a time of life when it is common to suffer loss and changing life circumstances. Moving from a house into an apartment or retirement community, giving up work or in some cases taking on new work, and facing the inevitable deaths of family members and friends are common challenges that occur during a woman's wisdom years. Since women live an average of 7.8 years longer than men, being widowed is a reality for many of us in our seventies and eighties. Some women respond to widowhood with resiliency, like Julia, and apply what they have learned to helping others. As a direct result of Roger's death, for instance, Julia added a conscious dying component to her elder program, both so that elders could assist the dying and so that they could come to terms with their own mortality in a way that facilitated the reality that death is the final process of growth rather than a time of deterioration and failure. The grandmother of a friend of mine was also a resilient elder. Sixty-eight when her husband died, she went back to college and earned a degree in archaeology. My stepdaughter's grandmother was in her midseventies when her husband passed away, leaving her with a forty-year-old son with Down's syndrome, who lives at home. She continues to be a pillar of strength, managing the apartment building that she owns, doing charitable work in the community, and helping out her granddaughter by providing child care for her great-grandson.

My father repeatedly counseled me to marry a man ten years younger so that I wouldn't be alone as I aged. Although I didn't do so, it was sound demographic advice. Almost 12 percent of the total female population are widows, compared to just under three percent of men, a statistic that mirrors our relative longevity. Once a woman is widowed, she can expect to live another seventeen years, often without male companionship, since the pool of available men is proportionately small. Statistics gathered in 1992 indicated that 34 percent of women between the ages of sixty-five and seventy-four lived alone. Half of women aged seventy-five and over lived alone and less than one quarter lived with a husband. The story is quite different for men. Even after the age of seventy-five, over two thirds of men live with a spouse.

Nature has been kind to men in terms of women's relative longevity, because when it comes to both psychological and physical resiliency after the loss of a spouse, men are the weaker sex. A large body of research documents the fact that illness and death increase significantly for widowers in the six months to two years after they lose a spouse. There is no such increase for women. Betty Friedan believes that women are more resilient because of a lifetime of practice in adapting to different roles. Another reason may relate to our lifelong penchant for connectedness. Women are traditionally the "kin keepers" who manage the social and holiday calendars and keep in touch with friends and relatives. A large number of studies have shown that social connectedness is an important buffer against all kinds of stress and loss, including bereavement. And while the number of people you feel connected to is important, the quality of the connection is even more important. Can you count on that person for help? Can you share your feelings with that person? Men are not only more prone to be loners, with few good friends, they have also been socialized not to share their feelings with other men. Their wives often become their emotional keel and rudder, and without her, they are lost. The resultant emotional isolation that occurs subsequent to her death creates stress and loneliness. Psychologist Janice Kiecolt-Glaser and her husband, immunologist Ronald Glaser, from Ohio State University Medical School, found that lonely people have a significant drop in a type of immune cell called the natural killer cell (NKC) compared to those who feel socially connected. NKCs scour the body to seek out and eliminate cancer and virus-infected cells. So a relative lack of these cells may predispose to illness.

Psychologist James Pennebaker at Southern Methodist University in Texas found that having an outlet for feelings was crucial to immune function and health. Even the simple act of confessing one's traumas to a shower curtain (there was no one behind it) protected the health of undergraduates who were monitored for six months after the experiment. Writing about traumas in journals, as long as one's feelings were discussed as well as the facts, likewise resulted in better health and more active natural killer cells to patrol the body and eliminate viruses and cancer.

The natural tendency for women to discuss their feelings and seek support during the grieving process is protective to our health. After Roger's death, Julia found great comfort in reminiscing about her husband with family and friends. They were also there for her when she felt lonely, overwhelmed, or depressed, which are the natural initial responses to loss. When my father died, family and friends came to my mother's house for several evenings in a row to "sit shiva," a Jewish custom of mourning. For seven days, friends and family are supposed to sit with the bereaved person, allowing them to reminisce about their loved one and tell stories of their life together. The house is filled with food, with company, and with people who can bring comfort. There is profound wisdom in such old traditions. As I spoke to the people who sat shiva with us, each one told me something special about my father, often something I didn't know. These conversations allowed me to build a fuller picture of him than I had had from the single perspective of being his daughter. They invested his life, and my memories of him, with deeper meaning.

The meaning that we give to any crisis, whether it's having to move out of a cherished house to an apartment or nursing home, suffering financial reversal, losing a loved one, or becoming ill, makes a tremendous difference to how we cope emotionally and fare physically. Some people react to crisis with despair, hopelessness, and depression which many studies have correlated with poor health; others react to similar events with resiliency that allows them to find new meaning and go on with their lives. Psychiatrist Viktor Frankl, who survived four Nazi concentration camps, wrote that suffering minus meaning equals despair. Resilient people cope by finding some positive meaning in their suffering, whereas despairing people often feel victimized.

Psychologist Martin Seligman of the University of Pennsylvania found that pessimistic people, who tend to feel helpless, often blame themselves for difficult events, and also believe that life won't get any better because they are incapable of making things better. My mother was a pessimist who blamed herself for my father's death. Weakened by cancer, and fearful of further treatments that had produced disastrous changes in his personality, my father chose to end his life by jumping out of the thirty-seventh story window of their high-rise apartment building at three A.M. one summer's morning. My mother never forgave herself for being asleep at that time. In her mind, my father's death was not his choice. It was her fault for not being awake to watch over him. The result of this belief, of the meaning she gave to his death, was lasting despair.

We cope with the inevitable losses that late adulthood brings in the same way we've coped throughout our lives. Whereas my mother was a pessimist, Julia was an optimist. Psychologist Suzanne Ouellette, of the City College of New York, has studied optimistic, resilient people like Julia whom she dubs "stress hardy." The three defining attitudes of stress hardiness all begin with the letter C, hence they are called the three Cs: challenge, control, and commitment. When Roger died, living alone was a challenge to Julia, rather than a threat to the status quo. Although the loneliness was real, so were the opportunities for continued growth, contribution to society, and pleasure. Although Julia was aware that she had no control over Roger's death, she also recognized that her response to this new phase of life was under her control. She was also fortunate that Roger's death was expected. Even if we have no control over a loss, such occurrences are less stressful if we can predict when they are likely occur. When rats are subjected to shock, for example, those animals who consistently hear a buzzer ten seconds before the shock is administered develop fewer ulcers than rats who get no warning. The last of the three Cs that characterized Julia's attitude was commitment, which is defined as an overarching set of values that give meaning to life. Julia was committed to service, to helping people at the senior center, in Third World countries, and wherever the opportunity arose because this was the highest expression of her spiritual beliefs.

The combination of strong social support, plus an optimistic attitude that made Julia resilient and stress hardy, are potentially available to all women. The woman who finds herself unable to cope with the grief that late life losses can bring needs to find professional help that can not only support her, but also help her to examine her attitudes. A patient of mine by the name of "Beverly" was in her early seventies when she came to the Mind/Body Clinic for help in controlling high blood pressure. It soon became clear that elevated blood pressure was the least of her problems. Her husband, Mel, had died about eighteen months previously and she felt cut adrift. The bridge games they had played with friends were no longer open to her since they were a couples activity. And since Mel was no longer there to cook for, she lost the avid interest in gourmet meals that had helped organize her time. Beverly was sad and depressed when I first met her, reminiscent of a midlife woman used to staying home and caring for her family who suffers from empty-nest syndrome until she makes the transition to the next phase of life.

In our ten-week mind/body program Beverly learned techniques for reducing stress that included diaphragmatic breathing, eliciting the relaxation response, and reframing beliefs that were keeping her stuck. Was the extra time she had on her hands since Mel's death a problem or was it opportunity to do something new and interesting? Was the withdrawal of some of her old friends who related to her only as part of a couple solely a loss, or did it make room for friends with whom she could share life more deeply?

When the ten-week program was over, Beverly asked to volunteer for us, answering the phone, giving out information about clinical programs, and making appointments. She loved the work, the comradery, and the opportunity to learn more about mind/body medicine. She also had a flair for interior design and helped several of us with office "makeovers." The information and skills she had learned about emotional literacy and psychological growth were intriguing to her, and she began to look around the community for opportunities to continue her growth and expand her interests. She joined the local Jewish Community Center and signed up for courses both on mysticism and on grieving. About a year after we'd met, Beverly was helping facilitate grief groups and had gone away on several trips with other adventuresome seniors through the Elder Hostel program. Although she would never have her old life back, she was finding unexpected pleasures in a new life. "Would you believe I camped in the Grand Canyon?" she asked me, an impish grin on her face. "I never thought there was life outside of the Holiday Inn. It took three months to get in shape for hiking, but I've never been more fit in my whole life." Her blood pressure was down and her spirits were up as day by day she created a new life. Grief and loss, for Beverly, were a stimulus to growth and evidence of the fact that we can continue to develop psychologically, emotionally, physically, intellectually, and spiritually throughout the life span.

KEEPING OUR WITS ABOUT US

Beverly found that her intellect was sharper than ever. She loved being a student again, reading books about Jewish sages and then repeating their wise stories to friends and people who came to the grief groups she helped out with. She "loses" a word now and then, and gets frustrated from time to time when she can't remember a name that she knows as well as her own. But contrary to popular opinion, this kind of minor word loss is not a function of losing our brain cells, and thus our wits. Although neurons do continue to die as we age, most pruning of extraneous cells actually occurs in utero, before we are even born. By birth we have already lost 50 percent of our neurons, but no one mourns the fading capacities of the infant brain. In fact, when pruning fails to occur in the young brain, there is an increased instance of mental retardation because there are too many extraneous circuits, too much noise, just as when competing television channels come in at the same time and neither is adequately clear.

Why should a neurological process that leads to clarity in younger years become suspect as we get older? Lay people and researchers alike have been conditioned by the "aging mystique" to fear a progressive loss of cognitive, or thinking, function later in life. Yet, as Berkeley neuroscientist Marian Diamond has demonstrated, aging rats who continue to be stimulated by their environments actually develop new cortical pathways that enlarge their brain mass. As pruning progresses during the aging process, in concert with the development of new functional pathways, there is every reason to conclude that the mind of a healthy woman like Beverly or Julia will continue to come into sharper focus.

Naturally, what comes into focus depends on the well-worn pathways that we've used throughout life. If we have habitually turned to helplessness or revenge, we will progressively become more embittered. If our focus has been on love, learning, and service, like Julia, we will progressively develop our oracular wisdom and the compassion that is a natural outgrowth of empathy and interrelational thinking. We age as we have lived, bringing the strengths and weaknesses of a lifetime to the process. As Katharine Hepburn remarked in her eighties, "I have no romantic feelings about age. Either you are interesting at any age or you are not."

CURIOSITY, CONTROL, AND LONGEVITY

Harvard psychologist Ellen Langer and her Yale colleague Judith Rodin believe that people who stay engaged with life, and have control over their environments, stay healthier and live longer than those who don't. They tested their hypothesis in a nursing home by splitting the residents into two groups. One group was passively cared for by the staff. The other group was encouraged to make personal decisions about their schedules. In addition, both groups were given a plant. In the passive group, the plant was cared for by nurses, while in the take-charge group, the residents had to care for it themselves. Eighteen months later, those who had been given initiative were far more vigorous, happy, and healthy than the passively cared for group. In addition, only 15 percent of them had died, compared to 30 percent of the passive residents.

Part of the aging mystique, according to Langer, revolves around the erroneous assumption that old people are unable to do things for themselves, that they are incompetent. This, of course, is a self-fulfilling prophecy because when other people do things for us that we could do for ourselves, we lose the stimulation required to continue developing mentally. Langer applied her theory to memory loss, one of the most feared aspects of aging. She and her colleagues asked nursing home residents questions about how many residents and staff there were, how many names they knew, and when various social activities were planned. Rewards, in the form of chips redeemable for goodies, were given to one group while two control groups either got chips without any relevance to their answers or no chips at all. Those who were encouraged to remember showed better memory of all things, were more vital, and lived longer than the other two groups. Two and a half years later, only 7 percent of the experimental group had died compared with about 30 percent of the two control groups.

When we lack stimulation at any age, mental processes and the ability to create begin to deteriorate. And when we stop creating, life-force energy diminishes and depression sets in. The prevalent myth of aging states that we gradually lose function and finally die. But what if the loss of function, and the associated decline in vigor, turn out to be a societal mind-set that we could avoid? Langer's data suggests just that. Very small changes in the way that we relate to the aging process can increase longevity and facilitate the ongoing development of wisdom.

LONGEVITY: POSSIBILITIES AND PITFALLS

I have no doubt at all that the aging process, in terms of its degenerative aspects, can be substantially retarded by attitude, opportunities for service, continuing intellectual stimulation and good health habits. The market for longevity books is growing by leaps and bounds as the book-buying population ages. So is the use of hormonal supplements like DHEA (dehydroepiandrosterone) that has been touted as a veritable fountain of youth. Does it really delay the aging process, protect against cancer, or keep the vital organs strong? There's not enough research yet to comment definitively on its benefits and potential liabilities, but there are some interesting theories and caveats.

DHEA is the most common and abundant of the steroid hormones (other steroids include cortisol, the estrogens, progesterone, testosterone, and aldosterone, which helps regulate sodium and potassium balance, and thus blood pressure). It is also a precursor, or building block, from which many other steroids including testosterone and the estrogens are synthesized. Therefore, a decrease in DHEA results in decreases in all the other steroid hormones. It has a host of functions in its own right, one of the most important being a substantial factor in tissue growth and repair. Its reparative capacities may indeed help restore certain functions, like immunity, that decline with age. Since

DHEA levels are highest in young adulthood, and decrease thereafter, it has been theorized that the decrease in DHEA is related to an increase in age-related degenerative diseases like arthritis, cardiovascular disease, and diabetes. Although the theory may turn out to have merit, there is still considerable research to be done, and much of what has been published pertains to men, rather than to women.

Dr. John Lee, a physician whose interest in the use of natural progesterone to relieve PMS and menopausal symptoms has led him to a careful inquiry into the intricacies of steroid synthesis and the biological effects of hormones, cautions against the use of DHEA for women since its role in breast cancer is unclear. He cites data that implicate low DHEA levels in breast cancer premenopausally, and high levels postmenopausally. Furthermore, DHEA inhibits the growth of breast cancer in normal mice, but stimulates breast cancer growth in mice whose ovaries have been removed and are therefore estrogen deficient. It is clear that more research on DHEA is needed, and also that effects on women must be distinguished from those on men, before the question of DHEA's safety and efficacy in ameliorating the degenerative effects of aging are known.

The best research on reversing the effects of aging involves the cardiovascular and immune systems, and confirms the fact that a healthy lifestyle and relaxation training can help keep the body functioning optimally.

The incidence of heart disease in women begins to creep up postmenopausally, peaking in the last quarter of life. More women die of heart disease, in fact, than die of breast and lung cancer combined. Physician and researcher Dean Ornish, author of *Dr. Ornish's Program for Reversing Coronary Artery Disease*, has published numerous articles in peer-reviewed scientific journals on the use of an ultra-low-fat vegetarian diet, stress management, meditation, yoga, and social support in the *reversal* of coronary artery disease. Sophisticated studies before and after going through his program show that arteriosclerotic plaques actually decrease in size, and in some incidences disappear entirely. Old arteries literally become young again.

Once again, social support shows up as an important factor both in the genesis and treatment of cardiovascular disease. Epidemiologists did a careful study of a town called Roseto, in Pennsylvania, because the residents had such a low incidence of cardiovascular disease. They were surprised that Rosetans were at normal risk for heart disease in terms of factors such as sedentary lifestyle, high-fat diet, obesity, cigarette smoking, and diabetes. They concluded that the social fabric of the community, which was unusually close and tight-knit, was the factor that reduced risk of heart disease. The most important value for Rosetans was time with family and friends. When researchers returned to Roseto twenty-five years later, however, heart disease was present at the same level as in the rest of the country. During those years the social fabric of the community had broken down. Children grew up and moved away in pursuit of the American Dream, searching for better jobs and more money. The remaining Rosetans began to be more concerned with consumer goods and less with connectedness.

Most of us are similar to today's Rosetans. You may recall that for busy working women in their thirties and forties, relationships with spouse and friends was a priority that lagged behind work and caring for home and children. When working women make the transition from a busy midlife, where social support often comes from people at work, to retirement, we may find that there is a void in our social support network. In the mid-1980s a psychiatrist from India was a visiting professor for one year at Harvard, where I got to know him. In 1989 I had occasion to visit India and participate in the first International Conference on Holistic Health and Medicine where he was also a participant. When I asked what his most lasting impression of America was, his answer shocked me. "It's the sad state of your women," he responded. He went on to say that women are by nature relational, that it is the core of our worldview and the foundation of our health and happiness. Yet most of the American women he met were so busy that they had little time for relationships. If, in our elder years, we don't replace the social support networks of our workplaces with other sources of friendship and mutual encouragement, research tells us that our physical hearts will suffer. I am convinced that part of the increase in heart disease that occurs in the last quarter of women's lives is indeed due to the relative isolation that many older women suffer from. The good news is that research like that of Dean Ornish demonstrates that whatever the cause of heart disease, social connectedness can help us renew the lining of our blood vessels and reduce our risk of heart attack.

The immune system, too, has the capacity to renew itself. Although immune function gradually decreases with age, no one has documented the actual reason for the decline. Is it preprogrammed genetically or is it secondary to the cumulative effects of lifestyle and attitude? As we have discussed, researchers at Ohio State Medical School found that lonely people have significantly lower measures of immune function than those who feel well connected. Immunity also takes a nosedive in those of us with poor coping skills, when we are faced with sudden stress as are many people later in life. But these effects are all temporary and easily reversible, as is the immunodepression that typically accompanies aging. Psychologist Janice Kiecolt-Glaser and her husband, immunologist Ronald Glaser, studied elderly people in nursing homes. One group was taught progressive muscle relaxation, a simple meditation exercise that shifts the body out of the stress response into the relaxation response, and a college student led them through it three times a week for three weeks. A second group was visited by students for the same amount of time, as a control for the possible positive effects of social support, and a third group received no intervention at all. At the end of just three weeks, the group who was doing the progressive muscle relaxation had a significant increase in two different measures of immune function, effectively restoring youthful measures of at least these two aspects of immune function. When they were asked to discontinue the practice, their immune levels fell to the starting point within just a few weeks. We still don't know if the immune rejuvenation was due to the physiological effects of the meditation, or whether it was a response to a new interest and an enhanced sense of control.

While I personally hope to live for a long time, I am uncomfortable with the implicit assumption of some authors that if we just do everything right, we'll automatically live to be a hundred. The accompanying, sometimes unstated, assumption is that if we die young, it is our own fault. This is a variation on what transpersonal psychologist Ken Wilber calls New Age Guilt, the idea that if we get sick, or fail to cure ourselves with the power of our mind, we have done something wrong. I get passionate about this subject because it extends beyond psychology and biology to the spiritual, a second implicit assumption being that if we are spiritually evolved enough, sickness and age will pass us by.

While we do, indeed, have the power to retard aging and to live

healthier lives, eventually all of us will die, and some will die at relatively young ages in spite of psychological resilience, good social support, capacity to love, and enviable health habits. Adele Davis,
renowned for her approach to healthy living and organic cooking, died
from cancer in her sixties. More than one person I knew threw in the
towel at the news, and went out to drown their sorrow at McDonald's.
The odd thinking was, "Gee, she did everything right and she died anyway. Why bother?" As Janet Quinn stated, there is no Cosmic Under-
writer who issues guarantees. It is only fear that seeks guarantees where
none exist. Bernadette Soubiros, the fourteen-year-old girl who saw the
apparition of the Virgin Mary at Lourdes, died in her early thirties of
bone cancer in spite of an elevated spiritual life. Living a psychologically and physically healthy life is its own reward, and although statistically these factors can extend our lives, individuals are not statistics.
None of us knows when and how we will die, but if we are fortunate
enough to have lived until seventy-five, the average expected life span
for women in America, it is prudent to begin considering death as the
final phase of our growth.

THE AMERICAN WAY OF DYING: A CHALLENGE TO PHYSICIANS AND FAMILIES

In her book, *Mindfulness*, psychologist Ellen Langer tells the story of
her grandmother's death from a brain tumor that went undiagnosed
medically even though her grandmother had pinpointed the problem
intuitively. She kept talking to the doctors about a snake that was
crawling around in her head. They simply wrote her off as senile, however, rather than using the valuable metaphor as a clue to the diagnosis.

Harried health-care professionals too often ignore both the implicit
wisdom of elders and their explicit instructions for how they would
like to die. A 1995 study in the prestigious *Journal of the American Medical Association* documented serious shortcomings in communication
between seriously ill hospitalized patients and their physicians. In a
large study involving over nine thousand patients, only 47 percent of
all physicians were aware of which of their patients had asked not to be

resuscitated. Furthermore, even in some cases where the physician was aware of such a request, they acted against the patient's expressed wishes in the belief that they knew the best course of treatment.

One of the patients I worked with was a sad case in point. "Ramona" had contracted the HIV virus from her husband, a man who had had just one homosexual encounter before they were married. A case of pneumocystis pneumonia heralded her diagnosis with full-blown AIDS. Ramona was one of the women participants in an AIDS group that I facilitated in the mid-1980s, and she returned to the Mind/Body Clinic frequently over the next year to attend subsequent groups and lend her support to others. She was generally in good health, although her T-lymphocyte count was very low, and she was one of those exceptional people who used the nearness of death to become more appreciative of life. Everybody loved her and held out the hope that she would be a long-term survivor, or even have a spontaneous remission of the illness.

I had done such a good job of convincing myself that she was invulnerable that I was shocked when she was admitted to the hospital with pneumonia for the second time. She had told her physician clearly that she did not want to be put on a ventilator or resuscitated, and was prepared to die rather than suffer through a long, incapacitating illness. Like many women I have worked with, Ramona was not so much afraid of death as she was of a prolonged process of dying. Her room was filled with cards and flowers, and cassettes of her favorite music played continuously day and night, because they helped create an atmosphere of peace. I came into her room one morning to find the soothing sounds of the tapes replaced by the mechanical hiss of a ventilator. Her body had been chemically paralyzed with a drug called curare so that her own breathing would not interfere with the pumping action of the machine, and her eyes were taped shut since she was unable to blink. The room was filled with the unmistakable scent of animal fear.

Her sister sat by her bedside weeping as she told me the story of how Ramona had been attached to the breathing machine against her will, struggling and protesting. The doctor, hoping that this young woman might rally from the pneumonia if she could be supported through the crisis on a ventilator, had simply ignored her pleas that she be allowed to die a natural death. She did die forty-eight hours later, and to this day I remain convinced that the cause of her death was sheer terror.

Attempts to keep dying people alive often create terrible pain for the person, physically and emotionally, as well as considerable stress for the family. Furthermore, such heroic measures are a substantial drain on the national economy. My mother was terminally ill with emphysema and congestive heart failure when hospitalized for the last ten days of her life. A constant series of tests were performed, in spite of the fact that both she and the staff knew that she was dying and she had signed a DNR. A hospital's business is to monitor vital signs, try to sustain them, and do tests to find out what is wrong so that life can be preserved—even if the patient is dying and has asked not to be resuscitated.

The morning of the day that my mother died she started to bleed internally. Rather than keeping her comfortable and letting her visit with the room full of friends and relatives who had come to say their good-byes, she was whisked off to the bowels of the hospital, to the nuclear medicine department, for testing. They wanted to pinpoint the source of the bleeding. She disappeared at ten A.M., and when she had not returned by late afternoon, I was dispatched to find her. She was lying alone and frightened on a gurney in the hospital corridor because the nuclear medicine department was backed up that day. I asked the physician in charge to let her go back to her room. He refused at first, stating the hospital's position that they needed a diagnosis. My mother, ever the wise guy, piped up in her husky voice, "Diagnosis? I've been laying here all day because you need a diagnosis? Why didn't you ask me?" The doctor was looking perplexed. "I'm dying," my mother concluded. "That's your diagnosis." And to his credit, he let her go without the test.

My mother made an obvious point. Yet, in the strange service of diagnosis without a purpose, she and our family lost several of the most precious hours of our lives together. The days of testing prior to her passing also racked up a huge medical bill that Medicare—meaning all of us—had to pay. The problem with medicine is that it doesn't know when to quit, and part of the reason for that is defensiveness. Some grieving people sue on behalf of dying relatives, believing that only one more procedure, one more test, might have kept their loved one alive. In fact, it is often a patient's loved ones who demand that a DNR be removed from the chart and that heroic measures counter to their loved one's wishes be instituted.

Doctors David and Christine Hibbard, a family practice physician and psychologist team who practice in Boulder, Colorado, have devised a simple and remarkably effective way for patients, families, and doctors to communicate. They call it the Patient-Family-Physician Guide, and you can order a copy by writing to the address supplied in the Resources section. Chris, who is both a friend and colleague, explained that the guide was developed because of experiences in which a patient's wishes were not honored either because of poor communication with the physician or well-intentioned meddling on the part of family members. When a person's wishes about how they want to die are not honored, the Hibbards have not only observed the kind of needless pain and suffering that we have discussed, but have also become acutely aware of missed opportunities for psychological and spiritual growth during the dying process. If a family insists on denying that their loved one is dying, for example, it makes it hard for the loved one to discuss their fears and say their good-byes. Saying good-bye often leads to sweet reminiscences about the shared lifetime, and allows the dying person to pass on her wisdom. It also gives family members a chance to express their gratitude to the dying person, and to let her know what she has meant to them. I have witnessed what I consider miracles in this process, in which old grudges are let go, forgiveness is claimed, and the hearts of all concerned become more peaceful. The time surrounding death is emotionally supercharged, and opportunities to finish old business and come to a new level of understanding abound. This is the gift of conscious dying. It can convert a difficult time into a holy time.

Part of the introduction to the Hibbards' copyrighted guide reads, "Death is a part of life and all of us are going to go through that process at some time. Although our society shelters us from death, we need to acknowledge the role it plays, its beauty, to learn from it, and make the right choices. We feel there is a need for all of us to have a relationship with death that is not based on the fear that our current culture supports." Part of alleviating that fear is the knowledge that each of us has the right to die with dignity, surrounded by loved ones to whom we have made our wishes clear. The opportunity for thanking one another, forgiving one another, and finding new levels of meaning in the years that have been shared is facilitated when seriously ill patients discuss their wishes about the dying process as clearly outlined in the guide.

I remember a woman named "Grace" who attended the Mind/Body Clinic in the hopes that meditative and imagery techniques might help reduce the suffering of a chronic itch she had, secondary to dialysis for kidney failure. Grace was in her midseventies when we met, happily married for over fifty years and the mother of three children. She and her family had faced the fact that Grace's remaining time was short, and she felt that their conversations about her death, and how she wanted to die, had brought them closer.

Grace wanted to die at home, and her husband, Mathew, was frightened at first. Could he deal with her pain? What would it be like to see the person he loved most in this world dying? What if he didn't have the strength to keep her home, and felt pressed to have her hospitalized in spite of her wishes? Two of Grace's children lived nearby, and together the family discussed how they could support Grace and Mathew. They got involved with Hospice, and Mathew realized that considerable help would be available, particularly in seeing to Grace's medical needs. Once Grace refused further dialysis, the time of her "active dying" would be short, and both children volunteered to stay with their parents during this time, if necessary. The solidarity of the family was a source of strength to all of them, and Grace remains etched in my memory as one of the most loving, peaceful people I have ever met.

THE GIFTS OF GRIEF, LOSS, AND RESILIENCY

Shakespeare wrote, "In calm seas all boats alike show mastery in floating. Only in a storm are they obliged to cope." The wisdom years bring many storms; widowhood, loss of friends, changes of residence, loss or changes in jobs. These are usually viewed as the inevitable miseries of old age, rather than as opportunities to see what we are made of. The lifelong pessimist who responds to these changes with despondency can learn to become resilient. The woman who loses her husband can find that an entire new and exciting life opens up to her.

Perhaps the greatest gift of the wisdom years is a renewed understanding of how important a network of close friends is to our health, happiness, and longevity. The woman who feels isolated, either because she has recently retired and left her job friends behind, or because her spouse has passed away, has an important opportunity to reevaluate her circumstances and reweave herself into the web of life. Seventy percent of women are still healthy in their seventies, and can continue to grow psychologically, intellectually, and spiritually. Much active and vital life still remains. Even the awareness that death is a reality, not just for others, but for ourselves, is a gift. In coming to terms with how we want to die, the way that we are living may come into bold relief. Are there things I want to accomplish in my remaining time? What are the most important things I can do for myself and others? Am I in a rut? The nearness of death calls these questions and can lead to choices that can help us to create new and more fulfilling lives in our elder years.

13

AGES 77–84 AND BEYOND: RECAPITULATING OUR LIVES

GENERATIVITY, RETROSPECTION, AND TRANSCENDENCE

At eighty Julia is unmarried like 75 percent of the women in her age bracket. She is bothered by arthritis, particularly in the fingers of her left hand and in her knees, but is otherwise in good health as are two thirds of the women who live to be her age. She lives in a three-bedroom condominium on Boston's waterfront that she has shared with her friend Barbara, also a widow, for the past six years. Fifty-one percent of women between the ages of seventy-five and eighty-four live alone; 29 percent live with spouses; and 20 percent live with other people. Julia dates a man named Mike, a retired police officer who volunteers at the senior center that she directed until she was seventy-four, and still consults for several hours a week. Since there are only fifty-three men for every hundred women between the ages of eighty and eighty-four, she counts herself lucky to have a love life. She enjoys spending time with Mike, and their lovemaking is a welcome gift.

Mike is seventy-eight, and had a moderately severe heart attack at seventy-five. He would like to get married, but Julia prefers to retain her freedom, in part out of the fear that Mike will become incapacitated and she will end up being his caretaker. Women Julia's age are much more likely to find themselves being caretakers of ailing spouses than they are to be recipients of care. Seven out of ten caregivers are women—wives, daughters, or daughters-in-law. And as of 1982, 37 percent of men over sixty-five who needed care were attended to by their spouses. Women are more likely to end up in nursing homes, but even so, statistics for 1985 indicate that only forty-five women out of a thousand, or 4.5 percent of those over seventy-five, were in long-term care facilities. In general, if we are fortunate enough to live into our eighties, our health is fairly robust.

Economics may be another matter. Julia is fortunate because the money she inherited from Roger, her own pension funds and investments, and social security have left her financially secure. In contrast, over 25 percent of elderly women had incomes that placed them below the poverty line in 1991, and the majority of others were very close to it. Because of her good health and financial situation, Julia has been able to continue her lifelong community interests. She is on several boards of advisors concerning health care and children's issues, and she volunteers frequently at the senior center where she is still a paid consultant.

In many ways, Julia is an example of what developmental theorist Erik Erikson called "generativity." She continues to give birth to ideas, and to bring forth new ideas in others. She calls to mind other generative elders like the world-famous conductor, Nadia Boulanger, the first woman to conduct the New York Philharmonic Orchestra. Born in Paris in 1887, Nadia Boulanger died in 1979 at the age of ninety-one. By the age of ninety she was blind, but continued to teach music with the same passion, rigor, and enthusiasm that had marked her entire career. In her elder years she considered herself doubly lucky. Lucky to be alive, and lucky to be in the presence of young people whom she could inspire and who inspired her. Her devotion to excellence in all things brought out the best in her students. Her generativity comes alive in a reminiscence. "I remember the old woman who cleaned the floor in my place in Gargenville. She died a few years ago. Every day I think of her with the most profound respect and with greatest reverence. She was eighty years old. One day she knocked at my door and said, 'Mademoi-selle, I know you do not like to be disturbed, but the floor, it shines in such a way. Come and see.' Now I think of her always. In my mind, Stravinsky and Madame Duval will always appear before the Lord for the same reason. Each has done what he does with all his conscious-ness."

CONTINUING ADVENTURES INTO GENERATIVITY

The last part of the life cycle, like all those that came before, has its own specific challenges and gifts. Physically, the immune system of the older woman begins to fail. The immune system is what differentiates between self and "not-self," protecting her from infections and disease. As we age, the immune system has an increasingly difficult time dis-cerning not-self. Everything begins to look like self. Instead of perceiv-ing this as a problem, we can view it as boundaries becoming more porous, the individual beginning to encompass more than what she thought herself to be. The older woman becomes inclusive, universal, taking in all as her own.

If we meet the challenge of generativity, rather than giving in to its opposite, which Erikson saw as despair, we can finish out our lives by leaving a legacy that continues to support others long after we are gone. Nadia Boulanger left hundreds of students, who in turn, will in-spire many more, not only to excellence in music, but to excellence of heart. Her housekeeper, Madame Duval, left a legacy of inspiration in doing what may have seemed to be a petty task, polishing the floor, with total attention. Julia's involvement with the eldering project also left a legacy, and after retiring from it, she felt a need to continue cre-ating. The inspiration for her next project—a book of stories that would help women reclaim their strength—came from an unexpected source, a little book written by an Alaskan woman, an Athabaskan In-dian named Velma Wallis, who retold an old legend entitled *Two Old Women*.

This story concerns two pampered elders, eighty and seventy-five, who have allowed themselves to be coddled by their tribe, gradually forgetting their own strengths. One particularly harsh and frigid winter, the Alaskan wilderness failed to yield enough game for the tribe to survive. Weak, starving, and discouraged, the chief reluctantly decided to abandon the two old women to conserve precious resources needed to journey in search of better hunting grounds. Forced to fall back on their own resources or die, the pair remembered a river several days' journey into the Arctic where the fish and game had once been plentiful. Pushing themselves to their limits and beyond, tolerating frigid temperatures and near starvation, the two old women made the painful trek back to the river. There they found abundant small animals to trap, and spent the winter camping comfortably in their strong hide tent and sewing rabbit hides into more blankets, hats, and mittens than they could use. Sitting alone by their fire, the women retrospected their lives and extracted levels of meaning that had been unappreciated before.

During the following spring, summer, and fall they fished, trapped, foraged, and hunted, finding daily that their strength and vigor increased. They laid in an enormous cache of food, much more than they required for the following winter. Their former tribe, meanwhile, was wandering in a destitute condition, having been unable to find good hunting. Starved, threadbare, and freezing, the ragtag band finally arrived back at the camp where they had deserted the two women the previous year. Ashamed for their actions—which they believed had brought them bad luck—they sent a scout to look for the women, in case of the remote possibility that they might still be alive. When the scout did manage to track the old women to their rich camping grounds, he was amazed to find them in such good condition while even the tribe's best hunters had wasted away.

Initially afraid of a second betrayal, the old women were cautious, but gradually forgave their families and friends, grateful for the reunion. Thanks to the two grandmothers, previously abandoned as useless, there was enough food and clothing for all to survive until spring. New hope and courage was spawned by their extraordinary tale of courage and transcendence, and the tribe once more found the heart to endure. The legend of the two old women appealed to Julia because she was in a period of her own life when there is a natural tendency to reappraise, reflect, and look for patterns of meaning. What was life all about? What were the major themes that developed? How can we best appreciate and learn from the story of our life?

RETROSPECTION AND THE FINAL LIFE TRANSITION

We go through a series of transitions in life, during which we reexamine what has gone before. The first transition is at the end of adolescence as we begin to form what the late Yale psychologist Daniel Levinson called an entry life structure for early adulthood. He described a second transition at midlife during which we reflect on our early adult life, distill what is most meaningful and important, and then plan our life structure for middle adulthood. The third, or late life, transition, which occurs between sixty and sixty-five, involves another period of retrospection and planning for our elder years.

I believe that there is a fourth, and previously undescribed, transition that occurs in the eighties. Rather than planning the next phase of earth life, we begin to extract the meaning of our lifetime as a whole, wondering about spiritual concerns. Every transition revolves around the central question, "What have I learned and how will it serve me in the next phase of life?" Since the next phase of life is death, reminiscing often takes on a moral quality. On the whole, was I good or not? Did I use the opportunities presented to me? How might I have done or seen things differently? What was the purpose of this life, which seemed to pass so slowly each day, yet, in the end, passed as quickly as a blink of the eye? What do I believe about an afterlife and how will the way that I lived my present life affect it? While not everybody lives into their eighties when this type of retrospection naturally occurs, I believe that most people experience it when they discover that they have a potentially life-challenging illness, no matter when that illness may occur during the life cycle.

One day when I was visiting my mother, who was eighty at the time, she told me that she'd been thinking back on her life and was sorrowful because of all the times she had been small-minded and judgmental. Since I had never known her to introspect and ponder psychological questions, I was surprised to find that she was not only reviewing her behavior, but questioning its roots. Why was she sometimes judgmental? Where did that behavior come from? It was not a way that she wished to remember herself. These were poignant questions for my mother. About a year later, when she was hospitalized just prior to dying, her retrospections and questioning took on a more overtly spiritual nature. She wondered about heaven and the possibility of an afterlife. She wanted to know if I believed that her parents and my father would be on the other side, waiting for her. And she wanted to make peace. In one short elevator ride from the basement, where she had been waiting for a test, to the seventh floor where her room was, we forgave one another. With great simplicity and directness she looked at me and said that she knew she had made many mistakes. Could I find it in my heart to forgive her? And in that moment, the misunderstandings and anger of a lifetime evaporated. I was also able to admit the many mistakes I had made, and to ask her to forgive me. In that holy moment when there were no barriers between us, I pressed my luck. I asked her to exchange a soul quality with me. Not normally the sort of person to whom that would have made sense, in her heightened state of spiritual awareness, it apparently made perfect sense. Without missing a beat, she told me that she admired my compassion and asked me to gift her with it. I, in turn, asked for her courage. This is the kind of psychospiritual growth and transcendence of past problems that can occur in the fourth transition, the final period of growth.

AN ATTITUDE OF GRATITUDE

My aunt Bertha is in her early nineties at this writing, still active despite a broken hip in her late eighties from which she recovered in time to dance at her grandniece's wedding. I have enjoyed hearing her retell the stories of her life. She has no regrets, having edited out all her problems by focusing on the things she is grateful for. In her own unassuming way, Bertha models an important psychospiritual process. When we focus on the good things in life, the things that we are thankful for, bitterness fades away. The Benedictine monk David Steindl-Rast wrote a luminous book entitled *Gratefulness, The Heart of Prayer*. He has found that if he can think of one thing to be grateful for each night that he has never been grateful for before, it makes him more mindful, aware, relaxed, and positive throughout the day. Bertha does this naturally. She reminds me of a little Jewish leprechaun, smiling as she retrospects and tells her stories of gratitude.

One of her favorite stories concerns the famous Coconut Grove fire in Boston. The Coconut Grove was a popular nightclub to which my parents often went with Bertha and her husband. One week Bertha was put in charge of making the reservation. Although she is a meticulously responsible person, for some incomprehensible reason, she just forgot to call the club. When Saturday night came, and my parents arrived, they were shocked to find that they had no reservations and had to go elsewhere. Bertha always laughs when she recalls how miffed my mother was. But not for long. Later that night, the Coconut Grove caught on fire and hundreds of people were killed either by the flames or in the ensuing stampede. It was one of Boston's worst tragedies. From the perspective of age, Bertha now believes their appointed time to die hadn't come, so a good angel had simply blocked her from remembering to make reservations.

Throughout the life cycle we consciously and unconsciously edit the events of our life, trying to give them meaning. We have all made mistakes, hurt others and been hurt ourselves, and through our difficulties, learned about life. What have we learned? What is most important? During the years that I worked in hospitals, I often did consultations for inpatients and would walk through the corridors where old patients often sat outside their rooms in wheelchairs. I was sometimes stopped, particularly by older women, who, due to a lifetime of relationality, are often gregarious as elders. If I had time, I would sit down for a while because these conversations were often profoundly interesting. There's an unusual quality I've noticed about many older women, a kind of transparency. It's as if they no longer have anything to prove, or anything to hide, so they are fully present. They have become like children again, with a kind of innocent directness.

One woman, whom I would estimate to have been about ninety, told me the story of emigrating from Ireland to Boston as a young girl. She married at nineteen and bore five children before her husband was killed in a railroad accident. She went to work as what used to be called a charwoman in a downtown business, eking out barely enough money to feed her family. But their life was full of love. The story she told was not one of bitterness, but one of human kindness, recollecting the many people who had helped her family through hard times. For her, the meaning of a life well lived was compassion and community. When

I left her and returned to my office, I tried a little harder to see every interaction as an opportunity for compassion. She had passed on her generativity to me.

STORIES AND THE QUEST FOR MEANING

The need for an older woman to tell and retell the stories of her life is no idle preoccupation with the past. It is a vital process of coming to terms with events and experiences in a way that can ultimately place them in an expanded frame of reference, giving the drama of a lifetime a cohesive, spiritual meaning. It is also a way for her to pass on wisdom to those who are younger. Great poetry and literature often derives its power from spiritual themes, as do contemporary movies. In Wordsworth's poem *Ode. Intimations of Immortality*, he piques the reader's interest with the line "Our birth is but a sleep and a forgetting: The soul that rises with us, our life's star, Hath elsewhere its setting." Moviegoers thrill to themes like that of *Ghost*, in which the spirit of the murdered Patrick Swayze stays near his lover, Demi Moore, in order to protect her. Only after she is safe does he travel up a beam of light into a heaven that the viewer is left to imagine. In the movie *Defending Your Life*, the newly deceased Meryl Streep undergoes a life review with a panel of angels in Judgment City. Her compassion and courage make her a shoo-in for heaven. A young man who is also undergoing a life review, and has not been able to overcome his fears and make the most of his potential, falls in love with her. When he finds out that he will have to be recycled to earth for another try at overcoming his fears, he becomes despondent about being separated from his new love. In a daring last-minute act of courage, he leaps from his own departing train and jumps onto hers. This act of courage, a repentance of his former cowardice and tendency to pass up opportunities, is enough to convince the angels that he is ready to go on with Meryl.

Both personally and collectively as a culture, we hunger for stories of spiritual meaning that will put the inevitable joys, sorrows, and frustrations of a lifetime into a meaningful context. In past times, Creation stories and stories about how human beings were supposed to act were told around the fire. Traditionally, it was the elders who passed on this wisdom. Neuroscientist Marcel Mesulam, of Northwestern University in Chicago, is intrigued by the fact that blood clots and small strokes preferentially affect the short-term memory of elders, which is mediated by the hippocampus, while long-term memory is spared. The person can still tell stories from the past, which Mesulam believes is an important function of later life. Neuroscientist and psychiatrist Mona Lisa Schulz, from the Maine Medical Center, interprets these findings in terms of the body's wisdom in preserving vital functions. For example, when a person hemorrhages, blood flow is shunted to the brain and kidneys to protect life. Similarly, neural circuits are wired to preserve the ability to tell stories, even after strokes or some forms of dementia have disrupted short-term memory.

An elderly relative of mine is a case in point. Now in her nineties, she began to suffer short-term memory loss sometime in her seventies. At a family gathering when she was in her late eighties, she went off to take a nap. When she awakened and rejoined the party, her face erupted into an enormous grin. "How did this happen, how did I get here?" she wondered aloud. "All the people I love are here." She then began to recount stories of that love. She took me back in great detail to my teenage years, during which I aspired to be a beatnik. I grew my hair long, wore dangling earrings and haunted the coffee houses in Harvard Square where I listened to, and sometimes played, folk music. My mother was horrified at my appearance and interests, but Esta championed my budding creativity both in dress and in music. An artist herself, she accompanied me to Harvard Square and bought me a fringed shawl that I still have. It has always been a symbol of self-expression, and a bond of love with a woman who encouraged me to be myself.

Hearing the stories of our escapades in Harvard Square, I realized how important it was for older women to mentor younger ones, encouraging them to find their talents. Esta's short-term memory was gone, but she was a true elder, telling the stories that helped the younger members of the tribe remember what was most important. From the beginning of time, elders have been the repository of tribal wisdom, and have handed down instructions about how best to live through the medium of stories. Some of these stories, which began as oral tradition, were eventually codified into sacred texts that provide transcendent spiritual meaning, an elevated context in which to understand the stories of our lives.

Native American teachings have remained in the oral tradition, handed down by elders from generation to generation. Vickie Downey is a Native American elder of Tewa descent, living at Tesuque Pueblo in New Mexico. She had a great deal to say about the oral tradition of stories, women, hidden wisdom, and the changing times. "In the beginning were the Instructions. We were to have compassion for one another, to live and work together, to depend on each other for support. We were told that we were all related and interconnected to one another. Now people call our Instructions legends because they were given as stories. But to the Indian people, that was like a reality at some point in history."

THE GIFTS AND CHALLENGES OF OLDER ADULTHOOD: A STORY OF DEATH AND REBIRTH

Throughout our tour of the feminine life cycle, I have frequently used stories to illustrate the challenges and gifts of each seven-year cycle, and the quadrant of life into which that cycle fits. My favorite story of generativity and transcendence, the gifts of the final cycle of life, concerns my mother, who was eighty-one when she died. A woman of prodigious strength who was embarrassed by emotions, her greatest fear was that if we dwelled on life's dark passages we would be overwhelmed by grief and give in to despair. "Ignorance is bliss" was her motto, and although it got her through life, my own path was very different. Whereas she looked away, I looked within. Whereas she lost faith when many of her family died in the Holocaust, the same event led me to quest for faith. Whereas psychological inquiry was folly to her until the last year of her life, it was the stuff of growth to me. In short, we were polar opposites who, at times, drove one another crazy.

The night of her death my son Justin, then twenty, and I were sitting on opposite sides of her bed meditating. I suddenly felt a kind of internal shift, as if my attention was being focused on a different level, and then I had a vision. I don't believe that it was a dream, because it felt like awakening to an expanded reality in which this life appeared to be a dream. In the vision I was a pregnant mother giving birth, and I was also the child being born. Conscious of being in two bodies at once, I had a deep knowing that all people are interconnected, a part of one another. Both mother and child were enduring a dark night of the soul, a deep pain that was the harbinger of rebirth.

Then my awareness slipped exclusively into the child being born and I found myself propelled down a long dark tunnel. I emerged into a kind of living light with the same characteristics described by people who have had near-death experiences. The light—a kind of formless divinity—exuded total love, bliss, wisdom, and mercy. I felt as if it had seen to the very depths of my soul and found me pure in spite of the many mistakes I had made in forty-three years of living. The purity, I was told, was a result of repentance—my attempt to learn from my mistakes. I was then told many things about the relationship my mother and I had shared, and every trial and difficulty seemed to have a higher purpose. At that moment I realized that our lives together had come full circle. My mother had birthed me physically into this life and I had just birthed her soul back out of it, and had been reborn myself in the process.

When I opened my eyes, the entire room seemed made of light, of energy. There were no boundaries between things. My mother's body was an energy form that graded into the air, the floor, the bed, the body of my son whom I saw weeping, a look of awe on his face. Justin looked at me with soft eyes and asked if I could see that everything was made of light. I nodded, and moved around the bed to sit next to him. He looked deeply into my eyes, and said, "This is Grandma's last gift. She's holding open the door to eternity so that we can have a glimpse." He went on to say that I must be very grateful to my mother for the gifts she had given me. When I nodded, he related some of the revelations he had received in that moment when the doorway between the two worlds temporarily opened. He told me that he understood that his grandmother was a wise soul, a very great being, and that she had displayed much less wisdom in this life than she actually had. This was part of our combined destiny, he continued, for in order for me to come more fully into my own life purpose I needed something to resist, to push against, so that I could become more fully myself and then share what I had learned with others.

There is an old Navajo saying that when we look at our lives from the earth side, it's like seeing the bottom of a rug. Unsightly threads hang down, and the pattern is confusing and unclear. But when we view our lives from above, as Justin and I did during my mother's death, we see a work of art woven from many strands, both dark and light, and we appreciate that all the threads were required to make the rug beautiful. Life is a gift, a work of art, and my hope is that this book has been an opportunity for you to appreciate the threads that make up the tapestry of the woman's life cycle in general, and an impetus to examine the threads of your own life in particular. Barbara Means Adams, a Lakota Sioux woman, wrote, "Every life is a circle. And within every life are smaller circles. A part of our lives goes full circle every seven years. We speak of living in cycles of seven." Let's look back over a summary of the feminine life cycle together now, in appreciation of the bio-psycho-spiritual gifts we have been given.

GIFT WRAPPING THE FEMININE LIFE CYCLE

Once upon a time an egg and sperm joined together in the timeless dance of fertilization. The egg, by nature nurturing and incorporative, enclosed the sperm within its substance and healed small injuries to its DNA that may have introduced unwelcome changes into the blueprint of life. The DNA, from what had once been the egg, carrying information from the dawn of life within its mitochondria, guided the newly formed cell in the intricacies of development. After nine lunar months, during which the developing child responded to pulses of information from the rhythms of the earth, the moon, and the hormones of her mother, she was born on a full moon, a beautiful baby girl.

The sight and smell of the child caused the mother's pituitary gland to release the hormone oxytocin, which both caused her uterus to contract and close off the blood vessels that had nourished the placenta, and coaxed her breasts into letting down colostrum, the first nourishment that her baby would receive in the outside world. The oxytocin also stimulated feelings deep within the mother's limbic system, or "emotional brain." She became totally infatuated with her newborn, doting on every movement, every look. It was love at first sight, a biological gift that eased the stress of the sleepless nights, fatigue, and inherent frustrations of caring for a newborn.

After several weeks, the baby began to smile and coo, and another kind of bonding began. Baby smiled, mother smiled. Baby cooed, mother cooed. It was as if the two were one. As the mother, father, or other caretakers mirrored the actions of the baby, the baby's nervous system began to myelinate pathways that extended from the emotional centers of the limbic system to the frontal lobes, the "heart of the brain." These circuits allowed the baby to attune more closely with her mother and others, reading the emotion in their faces, and mirroring their feelings to such an extent that the child could actually feel the same feelings. By eighteen months of age, the little girl's neural circuits for empathy were firmly in place. She had received the precious gift that would allow her to relate to others with compassion.

The little girl continued to mimic the characteristics of empathy and tenderness modeled by her mother and other women, developing a sense of self that is based on relationship to others, rather than independence from others. This way of relating to the world through "self-in-relation" provides a context in which two people can grow through a kind of mutual encouragement in which something emerges in relationship that is greater than the sum of its parts. But the little girl's growing sense of self-in-relation extends beyond other people to her relationship with the world at large. The girl child who has grown up in an emotionally healthy environment is a natural mystic. Like the poet William Blake, who wrote of seeing a world in a grain of sand, she is capable of perceiving the intricate web of interconnectedness that exists in an Oreo cookie. The rain and sun that grew the grain and cocoa, the harvesters and bakers, the shippers and stockers of shelves, and the little boy who gave her the cookie are intimately connected. She intuitively understands that nothing exists in isolation and that all of life is interdependent.

The intuitive, holistic thinking of the little girl is one of life's greatest gifts, an innate spirituality that informs a morality that takes many different viewpoints into account. Since the little girl has been socialized to play make-believe, the right hemisphere of her cerebral cortex develops a special richness of connections that preserves what Freud called "primary process" thinking, the kind of thinking that imbues even inanimate objects with spirit. This makes the little girl a keen observer who can use not only her eyes, ears, and logic, but can perceive deeper relations between things that she "knows" without knowing how she knows. This intuitive logic of the heart is a gift that allows her to understand the world as a complexity of intricate relationships.

Vocal and honest, the girl in middle childhood verbalizes what she knows. She has a kind of oracular gift that cuts beneath pleasantries and masks. Seven-year-old Brie, the daughter of a friend of mine, for example, asked pointed questions about my divorce and new relationship that many of my women friends were too embarrassed to voice. "What happened after twenty-five years of marriage? You're already dating a new man? Isn't it too soon? Don't you have to grieve for Miron and the life you shared first?"

Ebullient and self-assured in middle childhood, at around eleven the young girl begins to take certain societal injunctions seriously. It's not nice to be so outspoken. It's not ladylike. Don't be so smart or boys won't like you. The frontal lobes of the brain myelinate these injunctions into place, creating a database of socially acceptable behaviors, and the little truth teller begins to lose her voice. At about the same time, the powerful physiological changes of puberty are beginning, changes that are often accompanied by vivid dreams that were considered gifts of spirit in indigenous cultures, instructing the young girl in her life purpose. The pineal gland, sensitive to cycles and seasons, light and darkness, begins to send messages to the pituitary. Pulses of follicular stimulating hormone (FSH) and luteinizing hormone (LH) instruct the ovary to ripen eggs and prepare the uterine lining for a possible pregnancy. Estrogen and progesterone are produced, changing the contours of the adolescent body into that of a woman who becomes entrained to the lunar cycles. The young girl is then gifted with a deeper relation to her emotional life. In the first part of the menstrual cycle, when estrogen is high, she is outgoing and creative. In the second part of the cycle, under the influence of progesterone, she is more reflective. Just before her period comes her hormonal rhythms break through whatever veils the truth, and she may find herself brooding over problems. Neuropsychological testing shows that women hear fewer positive words premenstrually. When seen rightly this hormonal housecleaning, which is often called PMS, is a biological blessing meant to alert us to things in our life that may be blocking our happiness and creativity.

The teen years, in American society, may seem less of a gift than in indigenous cultures because the intuitive relational wisdom that strives to tell the truth, creating and restoring good relations, is opposed by Western culture that devalues these gifts. To be successful, the teen is told to embody the more masculine values of independence and autonomy, to be more wily and keep things to herself. She may even try to adopt the thin, hard-bodied physique of a man, popular in a culture where male versions of success have subtly infiltrated every aspect of life. But she cannot deny her innate relationality. Trying to find an identity, she gets stuck on the horns of a dilemma, "How can I be true to myself, without being selfish about the needs of others?" Resolving this dilemma, which Carol Gilligan posits as the central developmental task of adolescence, brings a tremendous gift. We realize the difference between selfishness and self-fullness. When we are self-full, true to our own perceptions, opinions, and needs, we don't have to worry about being selfish. We can depend upon our inherent compassion to do the right thing for all concerned. Even when our actions may disappoint others, we can see beyond the need to please people constantly, to the wisdom of allowing others to find their own strengths.

In my generation, very few women resolved the adolescent dilemma in adolescence. Many of us are still working through an understanding of our boundaries—where we begin and others end—in midlife. The healing of old wounds, the abuse and trauma that one-third of all women experience in childhood, must occur before we are emotionally healthy enough to maintain clear, compassionate boundaries and to live interdependently, rather than codependently as caretakers or counterdependently as isolated rebels. As the reality of emotional, physical, and sexual abuse has come to light, and as progressively more people have entered recovery programs for substance abuse, a new awareness of the importance of an emotionally healthy childhood has dawned. I believe that in future generations families will be better equipped to raise emotionally healthy children, and that more women will complete adolescent development in their late teens and early twenties, rather than in their late thirties and early forties when old issues of abuse and trauma seem naturally to arise for healing.

Throughout life we go through periodic transitions. The adolescent becomes a young adult. The young adult matures into midlife. Midlife gives way to the wisdom years. And the wisdom years give way to the mystery of death. Each time we move from one phase of life to the next, we engage in a period of retrospection and values clarification. What is most important? What is the measure of success? How can I be happy? At each of these transitions the feminine values triad of love, serenity, and service comes into sharper relief. The gifts of the feminine are also the gifts of health and longevity. When we are able to give and receive love, both the cardiovascular system and the immune system are more likely to function optimally. When we are peaceful the body can shift from the stress response to the relaxation response, bringing the body into homeostasis, or balance, and focusing the mind like a laser.

Each period of life transition has its own gifts. In our thirties we become aware of the war between two inner archetypes: Levinson's Traditional Homemaker Figure and the Antitraditional Figure. Can a woman only be happy in a traditionally female role as wife and mother? What are the pleasures and compromises of deciding on a career without children, or a career with children? How can we function in a predominantly male work world without sacrificing feminine values? The woman in her thirties today lives in a world very different than only a generation ago when the fledgling women's movement was just beginning to ask these questions. She has been gifted by the generations of women who came before her, and will leave a new legacy to the generation coming behind because she has been endowed with the understanding that her own masculine aspect is an ally, not a traitor. She doesn't have to fear that a successful career means abandoning relationality, because she knows that it is possible to balance masculine and feminine traits.

By her early forties transition, a woman is poised at the brink of a second puberty, another time of physical metamorphosis critical to her development as a woman. As adolescents we gain the physiological capacity to mother children. As midlife women we gain the capacity to nurture the larger world, beyond the boundaries of our nuclear family. The perimenopausal years of metamorphosis were previously viewed as a time when women lost sexual function and sex appeal, when we became less than we were. We are fortunate to be living in an era when, once more, there is a recognition that postmenopausal women have a unique role to play in society. Estrogen levels may be down, but testosterone levels are up. In midlife we become powerful forces to be reckoned with.

The blessings of midlife include a kind of fierce protectiveness of life, an intolerance for people and institutions that are selfish and out of accord with the values of relationality, and a powerful increase in the vividness of dreams and intuition. I have called the archetype of the midlife woman the Guardian because the wisdom and biology of a lifetime have come together in a way that supports her desire to protect the fragile, interdependent circle of life. Medical science treats menopausal women as tragic examples of estrogen deficiency, but new approaches based on natural and alternative medicine point out that we continue to make estrogen throughout our lives. As we tune in to the "symptoms" of menopause, they carry a powerful potential benefit of health. What is the effect of diet and attitude on our energy, hot flashes, dream life? Can we learn to use techniques of physiological self-regulation, like controlled breathing and meditation, in a way that not only makes the menopausal metamorphosis more comfortable but also helps protect our health and increases our peace of mind and creativity for the remainder of our lives?

The wave of the baby boom is now cresting in midlife, creating a population bulge of women who are the foundation of the 44 million Americans that sociologist Paul Ray calls Cultural Creatives (CCs). CCs are politically and socially active; believe in the feminine values triad of love, serenity, and service; and base their actions on the premise that all life is sacred, interdependent, and worthy of respect and preservation. As more women enter the midlife and wisdom years, this group, which already represents 24 percent of the population, will surely increase. Furthermore, younger women in their twenties and thirties are already heirs to the legacy that the women's movement—and the rise of interest in humanistic psychology and mind/body medicine begun in the 1960s and 1970s, and which informed the worldview of Cultural Creatives—has left for us all.

Women are coming into power and social consciousness earlier and earlier as the gap between generations closes and age distinctions blur. I find myself learning from women in their twenties, and from friends in their seventies. Perhaps the most important gift of the feminine life cycle is the gift of one another. As our lives become progressively busier, the message of caution that we have seen repeated in the research studies is that a woman's friends and, if she is married, her relationship with her spouse, are likely to take a backseat to family and career, at least through midlife. Isolation is difficult for any human, whether male or female, but for a woman it is what psychologists call "ego-dystonic," or out of tune with our accustomed way of being. For that reason, it has the potential to be a serious stress, and despite the busyness of our lives, we need to be mindful of the continued need to support and be supported by one another.

As we enter the elder wisdom years, time is once again available for friends, not just those of our own age, but those of every age. Sharing our wisdom with other seniors is wonderful, but sharing it with younger women and men is critical for the continued emotional, intellectual, political, spiritual, and moral development of our culture. Perhaps in the future the practice of isolating seniors in apartment complexes meant for elders only will be seen as a mistake. Throughout the life cycle we need to learn from one another and grow together if we are to bring about a new Integral Culture based on the feminine values of respect, interdependence, and care for future generations.

Appendix of Meditation and Prayer Practices

These ten simple practices can help reduce stress, bring about positive physiological changes that favor healing, and bring you into an awareness of wisdom. It is ideal to practice once or twice a day, for a few minutes at first, gradually working up to twenty minutes (or more if you like) each time. Many people find mornings a good time to practice, before the day gets going. It is also good to meditate before eating, since a big meal can make you sleepy.

While the exercises presented are best learned with eyes closed (unless specified otherwise), you can practice the breathing exercises with open eyes during the day while walking, doing the dishes, or waiting in line, even if you have only a minute or two. It's amazing what a moment of awareness and relaxation can accomplish. There are many types of meditation, and it's good to try several until you find one that comes naturally to you.

Don't worry if your mind wanders—everybody's does. The important thing is to maintain a relaxed but focused attitude, catching your-self when you are thinking, and letting go of the thought as quickly as possible, returning to the exercise. All of these meditations and more can be found in my book of daily meditation, inspiration, and prayer, *Pocketful of Miracles*, from which this Appendix was adapted. If you prefer to meditate using audiotapes, you might enjoy ordering those that I have prepared. There is a listing in the Resource section.

Exercise 1: Belly Breathing

Awareness of breath is the cornerstone for developing control of the body/mind. When the breath is shallow and fast, the body responds with an increase in heart rate, blood pressure, and fear hormones. The mind responds with fantasies of loneliness, unworthiness, and negativ-ity. When the breath is long and slow, the body becomes peaceful and relaxed. The mind stops churning and comes to rest. Normally we fo-cus on the inhalation, rather than on the exhalation, which is often in-complete. So in belly breathing, awareness is kept mostly on the exhalation, which is smooth and slow.

Close your eyes and become aware of your breathing now.....Is it shallow and irregular or deep and slow?.....Take a big breath in and let it go slowly, like a sigh of relief, focusing on releasing it completely. Let the next breath come in naturally and feel (or imagine) how your belly expands. When you exhale, feel (or imagine) how your belly re-laxes.....As you breathe from your belly, notice how both mind and body come to rest.

Exercise 2: Counting the Breaths

Close your eyes and take a letting-go breath, a big sigh of relief.....Now shift to belly breathing. On the next out breath, mentally concentrate on the number four.....On the next out breath, three, then two, then one on successive out breaths.....Start counting down from four again and continue for five minutes. Whenever thoughts come to mind, just notice them and let them go as soon as possible, returning your atten-tion to breathing and counting.

Exercise 3: Breath of Bridging Earth and Heaven

Meditate outside if possible when first learning this meditation. Sit with your feet solidly upon the earth, close your eyes, and begin with a minute of belly breathing.....Now place your awareness at the bottoms of your feet and either feel or imagine the energy of Mother Earth.....Breathe that energy into your heart and breathe out a sense of compassionate awareness.....Now either feel or imagine the energy of Father Sun shining down on you.....Breathe it in through the top of your head, taking it into your heart. Breathe out a sense of compassionate awareness.....Now breathe in the sunlight from above and the earth energies from below and let them meet and marry in your heart.....Breathe out the creative, loving energies of earth and sky that have been blessed by your being.....Let each out breath expand to caress all creation, continuing for as long as you like.

I practice this breath with eyes open many times during the day as I'm going about my business.

Exercise 4: Basic Concentration Meditation

Meditation is a form of mental martial arts. If we resist thoughts they will overpower us. But if we just step lightly out of their way, letting them come and go like birds flying overhead, we can use their energy to focus our minds further. Choosing a mental focus—a mantra or prayer word—is one of the oldest recorded types of meditation. The word is repeated on every exhalation. I enjoy using the expression "thank you," which reminds me to be grateful for the gift of life.

Close your eyes and take a big letting-go breath.....letting yourself slide into the relaxation of belly breathing. On every out breath, repeat a word, phrase, or short prayer of your choice. When thoughts arise, just notice and let them go, returning your attention to the breath and the focus word.

Exercise 5: Stretching

Mind and body are so intimately related that they form a "bodymind" unit. When the body is relaxed, the mind slows down. When the mind slows down, the body relaxes. Before meditation and throughout the day remembering to stretch the body allows the mind to be spacious. Before prayer and meditation, and throughout the day when you feel stressed or fatigued, take a moment to stretch.

Close your eyes and center yourself with your breath, becoming aware of the state of your muscles in your face, neck, shoulders, and back. Sometimes just paying attention helps to let go and relax.....Now inhale and gently arch your back, dropping your head back.....then exhale and round your back forward, dropping your chin to your chest.....Now inhale and stretch your arms above your head, placing the backs of the hands together, then exhale and let them float slowly down to your sides as if you were making a snow angel.....Next, gently drop your head toward the right shoulder, and then to left—back and forth several times.....Now repeat the motion, dropping your chin to your chest and then dropping it toward your back. Stretch your face with a big yawn.

Notice how your body feels two or three times each day. Then stretch and observe how your body and mind respond to the attention.

Exercise 6: Holy Moment Meditation

Close your eyes and take a few letting-go breaths. Now remember a time when you felt present in the moment—absorbed in a sunset, marveling at fresh-fallen snow, enchanted by the smile of a baby.....Enter the memory with all your senses.....Remember the sights and colors, the smells, the position and movement of your body, the emotions and the way that you feel those emotions physically.....as body sensations.....Now let the memory go and meditate for a few minutes on the feelings that remain.

Every moment that you are in the present is a holy moment.

Exercise 7: Centering Prayer

Centering prayer is a form of meditation that has been popularized by the Trappist monk Thomas Keating. It is based on practices written about by the third-century desert fathers of early Christianity. Keating's book on centering prayer, *Open Heart, Open Mind*, is a treasure regardless of what your religious orientation may be. Centering prayer is a very quiet meditation, a deep letting go to the inner silence, to the Mind of God. It is truly a resting in the Divine Presence. Keating compares awareness of our thoughts to boats that are floating down a river. Normally we are unaware of the river, which is God's Presence. He explains that centering prayer is a shifting of attention away from the boats to the river upon which they float. As in concentration meditation, you will choose a prayer word, although it is used very differently, and without an awareness of the breath. Rather than focusing on the word, you are focusing on the silent comfort and deep peace of God's Presence. The word is used only when the mind gets restless, helping you focus once again on letting go to the silence.

Begin by bringing back a holy moment as in the previous exercise, then let it go, focusing on the openhearted feelings that remain.....Now begin centering prayer, letting go to the deep peace of an open heart, God's heart.....When you begin to think, mentally repeat a word or phrase of your choice—a prayer term like *thank you, peace, shalom, kyrie eleison*.....As soon as your mind quiets down again, let go of the word, which is simply a reminder of your intention to sit quietly in the peace of God's Presence.

Exercise 8: The Egg of Light

Close your eyes and center with a few letting-go breaths. Now in the space above you imagine a great star of light.....Feel streams of Divine love and light flowing down over you, refreshing you, and then entering through the top of your head. Let this river of light wash through your body, the way that a river washes through the sand on its bottom, carrying away any fatigue, fear, or negativity.....As all the darkness washes out of the bottoms of your feet, let Mother Earth take it in and transform it.....As the light continues to wash through you, let it scrub clean the boundaries of your heart.....Now let your heartlight expand and fill your body.....let it move beyond the limits of your body for two or three feet in all directions.....above and below you, and all around, mingling with the Divine light from above and encasing you in a protective egg of light. Rest in the presence of the light for a few minutes, using any meditation that you enjoy.

Exercise 9: Loving-kindness (Metta) Meditation

Close your eyes and begin by taking a few letting-go breaths and then enter the inner sanctuary of stillness.....Imagine a great star of light above you, pouring a waterfall of love and light over you.....Let the light enter the top of your head and wash through you, revealing the purity of your own heart, which expands and extends beyond you, merging with the Divine light.....See yourself totally enclosed in the egg of light and then repeat these loving-kindness blessings for yourself.

> *May I be at peace.*
> *May my heart remain open.*
> *May I awaken to the light of my own true nature.*
> *May I be healed.*
> *May I be a source of healing for all beings.*

Next, bring a loved one to mind. See them in as much detail as possible, imagining the loving light shining down on them and washing through them, revealing the light within their own heart. Imagine this light growing brighter, merging with the Divine light and enclosing them in the egg of light. Then bless them.

> *May you be at peace.*
> *May your heart remain open.*
> *May you awaken to the light of your own true nature.*
> *May you be healed.*
> *May you be a source of healing for all beings.*

Repeat this for as many people as you wish.

Next, think of a person whom you hold in judgment, and to whom you're ready to begin extending forgiveness. Place them in the egg of light, and see the light washing away all negativity and illusion, just as it did for you and your loved ones. Bless them:

May you be at peace.
May your heart remain open.
May you awaken to the light of your own true nature.
May you be healed.
May you be a source of healing for all beings.

See our beautiful planet as it appears from outer space, a delicate jewel spinning slowly in the starry vastness.....Imagine the earth surrounded by light—the green continents, the blue waters, the white polar caps.....The two-leggeds and four-leggeds, the fish that swim and the birds that fly.....Earth is a place of opposites.....Day and night, good and evil, up and down, male and female. Be spacious enough to hold it all as you offer these blessings:

May there be peace on earth.
May the hearts of all people be open to themselves and to each other.
May all people awaken to the light of their own true nature.
May all creation be blessed and be a blessing to All That Is.

Exercise 10: Mindfulness Meditation

The Tibetan Buddhist practice of *shamatha/vipassana* means the "meditation of calm abiding and insight." It is a basic practice for seeing with the Wisdom Self, rather than through the eyes of the ego. Excellent instructions are given in *The Tibetan Book of Living and Dying*, by Sogyal Rinpoche.

Sit in your seat with great dignity, back straight and eyes open.....Look directly in front of you, eyes down slightly, without particular focus.....Or, if you prefer, close your eyes. Become aware of your breathing—how breath comes in and fills you and how breath moves out into space. Keep about one quarter of your attention on breathing and the other three quarters on the feeling of spaciousness. When thoughts arise, just let them go by.....

Sogyal Rinpoche, a Tibetan Buddhist lama, compares the thoughts that arise in meditation to waves that rise from the ocean. It is the ocean's nature to rise. We cannot stop it, but as Rinpoche says, we can "leave the risings in the risings."

Resources

- *Circle of Healing Newsletter and Catalogue*

Mind/Body Health Sciences, Inc.
393 Dixon Road
Boulder, CO 80302
(303) 440-8460 phone
(303) 440-7580 fax

Free annual publication featuring Joan's lecture and workshop itinerary, information on A Gathering of Women weekend spiritual retreats, her books, audiotapes, and videos, plus a select offering of healing music, art, and meditation tapes for adults and children.

- *Books by Joan Borysenko*

Minding the Body, Mending the Mind. Bantam Books, 1987. (basic meditation and psychological healing practices)

Guilt Is the Teacher, Love Is the Lesson. Warner Books, 1990. (healing the wounds of childhood and orienting to the spiritual self)

On Wings of Light: Meditations for Awakening to the Source; cocreated with artist Joan Drescher. Warner Books, 1992. (magnificent illustrations and meditations for humans from six to a hundred and six) There is also an audiocassette version of *On Wings of Light,* narrated by Joan, with an original soundtrack.

Fire in the Soul: A New Psychology of Spiritual Optimism. Warner Books, 1993. (a book for anyone going through crisis, grieving, or wondering about the age-old question of why suffering exists in a loving universe)

Pocketful of Miracles. Warner Books, 1995. (a book of daily spiritual practice, prayer, and inspiration)

The Power of the Mind to Heal; with Miroslav Borysenko. Hay House, 1995. (an update on the connection between mind/body and spirit)

- *Audiocassette Programs by Joan Borysenko*

Meditations for Relaxation and Stress Reduction

Meditations for Self-Healing and Inner Power

Meditations for Healing the Inner Child and Improving Relationships (for women)

Meditation on: Invocation of the Angels

Meditation on: Overcoming Depression

Meditation on: Loving-kindness and Compassion

Meditation on: Women's Wisdom at Midlife

Minding the Body, Mending the Mind. (Joan reads her classic *New York Times* best-seller, four-tape set)

The Power of the Mind to Heal. Nightengale Conant, 1993. (six double-sided cassettes that provide up-to-date medical and psychological knowledge about healing, enhanced by wisdom from the world's great spiritual traditions. The set includes several guided meditations and a set of inspiring prayer cards.)

Seventy Times Seven: On the Spiritual Art of Forgiveness (a three-hour program featuring wisdom and meditations drawn from Jewish, Christian, Taoist, and Native American traditions)

A variety of lecture tapes on topics that range from spirituality, to psychology, women's issues and mind/body healing.

- *A Gathering of Women Retreats*

c/o Mind/Body Health Sciences, Inc.
393 Dixon Road
Boulder CO, 80302
(303) 440-8460 phone
(303) 440-7580 fax

Joan Borysenko, Elizabeth Lawrence, and Jan Meier invite you to join us for a weekend of spiritual renewal and sisterhood (Friday evening through Sunday lunch). We conduct these several times annually in retreat settings across the country and in Mexico. Prayer, meditation, song, and ritual drawn from a wealth of traditions create a sacred space and a time for deepening our connection to self, others, and the Divine Source.

Joan, Elizabeth, and other staff members are also available for retreats customized for your group which they can do together, alone, or in conjunction with other programs. Please call or write for further information.

- *The Inner Connection*

Elizabeth Lawrence, M.A.
P.O. Box 169
North Scituate, MA 02060

Please write for information on international "spiritual getaways"; corporate, hospital, or personal training in healing by the laying on of hands; and individual sessions in energy healing and the healing of memories.

- *Women of Vision Network*

c/o Barbara Webber
P.O. Box 522
Bowie, MD 20718
(310) 805-WVWV (9898)

An organizing principle of this group is that "The feminine, which has been submerged for many years, is finally coming forward. It is time for woman to take her rightful place, not to dominate man, but to join with him in partnership for a better world. It is time for us to take action to shape the kind of world we want for ourselves, our children, and all future generations." Women of Vision was born out of a 1991 meeting in Washington, D.C., where participants from the United States and the Middle East gathered to discuss leadership for a new world. Since then, many regional conferences have been held, and policies developed in areas as diverse as religion, government, ecology, economy, health care, education, human rights, and the media. Please join in creating a better society!

• *Dr. Christiane Northrup's Health Wisdom for Women Newsletter*

Phillips Publishing, Inc.
7811 Montrose Road
P.O. Box 60110
Potomac, MD 20897-5924
(800) 804-0935

A provocative monthly newsletter focusing on natural healing alternatives, and the role that emotions play in heath.

• *Women's Health Advocate Newsletter*

P.O. Box 420235
Palm Coast, FL 32142-0235
(800) 829-5876

This monthly newsletter is an excellent publication, produced by a renowned panel of women physicians and scientists, which spans issues of public policy and personal health issues.

• *MidLife Woman Newsletter*

MidLife Women's Network
5129 Logan Avenue South
Minneapolis, MN 55419-1019
(800) 886-4354

This bimonthly newsletter targeted for women thirty-five to sixty-five years of age is packed with up-to-date information on health, psychology, and women's issues. Topics such as caring for aging parents, assessing the effectiveness of natural hormones, the controversy over hysterectomy, midlife career issues, and reports from worldwide conferences are clearly and responsibly covered.

- *Womankind Journal and Catalogue*

P.O. Box 1775
Sebastopol, CA 95473
(707) 522-8662

This catalogue was started by Tamara Slayton, an educator in menstrual health and women's cycles. It is filled with interesting quotes, books, items for rituals, and products like reusable cloth menstrual pads.

- *Institute of Noetic Sciences*

475 Gate 5 Road
Sausalito, CA 94965
(415) 332-5777

This quarterly journal explores the furthest reaches of what it means to be human, with articles by leaders in the field of consciousness research. It also has excellent book reviews and a fine mail-order catalogue.

- *Common Boundary*

P.O. Box 445
Mt. Morris, IL 61054
(800) 548-8737

This bimonthly magazine explores the boundary between psychology and spirituality. They have a comprehensive listing of conferences and programs occurring throughout the country, many of which are continuing-education opportunities in mind/body medicine and psychology.

• *The Healing Healthcare Network*

Kaiser and Associates
P.O. Box 339
Brighton, CO 80601
(303) 659-7995

The Healing Healthcare Network is an association of organizations committed to developing health care that heals as well as cures. The network publishes *Healing Healthcare*, maintains information resources on a variety of topics in the healing area, and operates HealthOnline, a computer bulletin board system, for individuals discussing healing and other health-care topics with national leaders.

• *The Lionheart Foundation*

c/o Robin Casarjian
P.O. Box 194
Boston, MA 02117
(617) 965-1215

The Lionheart Prison Project is dedicated to providing healing for prisoners and taking the first steps to transform prisons into "houses of healing." Robin is the author of *Forgiveness: A Bold Choice for a Peaceful Heart*, and *Houses of Healing*, a book for prisoners. She has brought these much-needed principles of healing into the criminal justice system. Please join us in supporting her work if you can.

• *The Humor Potential*

Loretta LaRoche, M.D. (Mirth Doctor)
15 Peter Road
Plymouth, MA 02360
(508) 224-2280

I have known Loretta for years. She is hands down the funniest wise-woman alive. She has offered programs to patients and staff of the Mind/Body Medical Institute in Boston and hundreds of other hospitals, schools, and businesses across the United States. Her humor helps us to see ourselves psychologically, overcome old habits, and really use the power of the mind to heal ourselves and enjoy our lives. Write or call for a free Humor Potential catalogue and help stop global whining!

- *Murals for Healing*

Joan Drescher
23 Cedar Street
Hingham, MA 02043
(617) 749-6179

Joan is an artist who has published over twenty-five children's book as well as cocreating *On Wings of Light: Meditations for Awakening to the Source* with Joan Borysenko. Her company provides both original murals and reproductions of her murals to hospitals and clinics seeking to create a healing environment. Write or call for a free brochure.

- *Janet Quinn, R.N., Ph.D., F.A.A.N.*

Therapeutic Touch: A Homestudy Course for Caregivers
This exceptional video can be ordered from:

The National League for Nursing
350 Hudson Street
New York, N.Y. 10014
(800) 669-9656

Janet has also created a uniquely beautiful set of WomanStones, sensuously handcrafted stones that fit into the palm of the hand inscribed with inspirational messages for women. They come accompanied by a booklet expanding on the theme of each stone. For ordering information please write to:

Dr. Janet Quinn
3080 Third Street
Boulder, CO 80303

- *Patient-Family-Physician Guide*

This valuable guide for families and physicians can help to insure a peaceful process of dying by stimulating a thorough inquiry into what medical/technical support a person would find acceptable in a variety of different circumstances. To order a copy, write to:

David Hibbard, M.D.
Family Medical Center
877 South Boulder Road
Louisville, CO 80027

Please include five dollars for postage and handling.

NOTES

INTRODUCTION
The Feminine Life Cycle

Page 2. . . . scant differences have been found between men and women. A. Fausto-Sterling, *Myths of Gender Biological Theories About Men and Women*, 2nd ed. (New York: Basic Books, 1992).

Page 4. Ancient Chinese philosophy, as described in *The Yellow Emperor's Classic of Internal Medicine*, employed a similar system of sevens . . . *The Yellow Emperor's Classic of Internal Medicine*, trans. I. Veith (Berkeley: University of California Press, 1972).

Page 5. Furthermore, if you live to be sixty-five, statistics predict that you can expect to live another 18.8 years—or until eighty-four. *The American Woman: 1994–95*, ed. C. Costello and A. J. Stone (New York: W. W. Norton, 1995).

Page 5. . . . the number of women between forty-five and fifty-four will increase by one-half (from 13 to 19 million) by the year 2000. G. Sheehy, *Menopause: The Silent Passage* (New York: Pocket Books, 1991).

Page 6. Only 17 percent of the population is over forty. *The American Woman: 1994–95*, ed. C. Costello and A. J. Stone (New York: W. W. Norton, 1995).

Page 8. "Woman is an unfinished man, left standing on a lower step in the scale of development." Aristotle, "Physics." In *Aristotle and the Earlier Peripatetics*, vol. 2, ed. B. F. C. Costelloe and J. H. Muirhead (London: Longman's Green and Co., 1897), p. 55.

CHAPTER ONE
Becoming a Woman: From Adam's Rib to Eve's Chromosomes

Page 12. ". . . the one gives the soul, the other the body." Aristotle, "Physics." In *Aristotle and the Earlier Peripatetics*, vol. 2, ed. B. F. C. Costelloe and J. H. Muirhead (London: Longman's Green and Co., 1897), pp. 49–50.

Page 13. The theories of gender development at the end of the 1800s were summarized in a British text entitled *The Evolution of Sex . . .* P. Geddes and J. A. Thomson, *The Evolution of Sex* (London: Walter Scott, Ltd., 1895).

Page 13. In the early 1950s a researcher by the name of Jost discovered that the normal course of human development is female. A. Jost, "Problems of Fetal Endocrinology: The Gonadal and Hypophyseal Hormones," *Recent Progress in Hormonal Research* 8 (1953): 379–418.

Page 14. In order for a male to develop, testis-determining genes on the y-chromosome must be activated to neutralize the ovary-determining genes. F. W. George and J. D. Wilson, "Sex Determination and Differentiation," chap. 1. In *The Physiology of Reproduction*, 2d ed., ed. E. Knobil and J. D. Neill (New York: Raven Press, Ltd., 1994).

Page 15. So in tracing the origins of mitochondrial DNA, biologists have also been able to trace our matrilineal family tree back to an African Eve . . . A. C. Wilson and R. L. Cann, "The Recent African Genesis of Humans," *Scientific American* (April 1992): 68–72.

CHAPTER TWO
Ages 0–7: Early Childhood
From Empathy to Interdependence

Page 21. . . . the "four Fs" of fighting, fleeing, feeding, and sex. J. Hooper and D. Teresi, *The 3-Pound Universe* (New York: Macmillan Publishing Company, 1986), p. 43.

Page 22. If a baby is born with cataracts that are not removed until the age of two, she will be blind for life. Research on critical periods of neural development is reviewed by S. Begley, "Your Child's Brain," *Newsweek* (19 Feb., 1996): 55–58.

Page 22. . . . newborn babies show a limited type of empathy by crying when they hear another infant in distress, a reflex called *motor mimicry* . . . The research on motor mimicry through infancy to the toddler years is discussed by D. Goleman, *Emotional Intelligence* (New York: Bantam Books, 1995), pp. 98–99.

Page 23. Only hours after birth the infant moves her body in a precise synchrony with the speech patterns of her caretaker. W. S. Condon and L. W. Sander. "Neonate Movement Is Synchronized with Adult Speech: Interactional Participation and Language Acquisition." *Science* 183 (1974): 99–101.

Page 23. . . . human faces are a baby's favorite sight, and human voices her preferred sounds. For an excellent description of early childhood and infant development, see Z. Rubin and E. B. McNeil, *Psychology: Being Human* (New York: Harper and Row, 1985), pp. 225–52.

Page 25. "Our conception of the self-in-relation involves the recognition that, for women, the primary experience of self is relational, that is, the self is organized and developed in the context of important relationships." J. Surrey, "The Self-in-Relation: A Theory of Women's Development." In *Women's Growth in Connection: Writings from the Stone Center,* J. V. Jordan, A. G. Kaplan, J. B. Miller, I. P. Stiver, J. L. Surrey (New York: Guilford Press, 1991), p. 52.

Page 26. . . . "this leads them to be more experienced at articulating their feelings and more skilled than boys at using words to explore and substitute for emotional reactions such as physical fights. . . ." D. Goleman, *Emotional Intelligence* (New York: Bantam Books, 1995), p. 131.

Page 27. In experiments done in pairs, when one person is in charge and the other is subordinate, the individual of lower status quickly learns to attend to the nonverbal cues of the "boss" no matter what their gender. C. Tavris, *The Mismeasure of Women* (New York: Simon and Schuster, 1992), p. 64.

Page 28. . . . "relationship authenticity," the "ongoing challenge to feel emotionally 'real,' connected, vital, clear, and purposeful in relationship." J. Surrey, "The Self-in-Relation: A Theory of Women's Development," p. 60. In *Women's Growth in Connection: Writings from the Stone Center,* J. V. Jordan, A. G. Kaplan, J. B. Miller, I. P. Stiver, J. L. Surrey (New York: Guilford Press, 1991).

Page 33. In the aboriginal Creation myth, Baiame (the creator) lay sleeping. C. Havecker, *Understanding Aboriginal Culture* (Sydney, Australia: Cosmos Periodicals Ltd., 1987).

Page 34. "He [Baiame] sent a message by clear sentience . . ." Ibid., p. 2.

CHAPTER THREE
Ages 7–14: Middle Childhood
The Logic of the Heart

Page 37. In comparison to boys, studies show that girls of this age are more resilient and optimistic . . . Research on gender differences in optimism at different ages is reviewed by M. E. P. Seligman, *Learned Optimism* (New York: Alfred A. Knopf, 1991).

Page 38. . . . to investigate the way in which the nervous system converts letters on a page into sounds. Although they were not looking for male/female differences . . . B. A. Shaywitz, S. E. Shaywitz, et al., "Sex Differences in the Functional Organization of the Brain for Language," *Nature* 373: (1995): 607–609.

Page 40. Other research data strongly suggests that gender plays no role in moral decision making. S. Callahan, "Does Gender Make a Difference in Moral Decision Making?" *Second Opinion* 17, (October 1991): 66–77.

Page 40. Piaget linked cognitive development to how we make moral judgments. J. Piaget, *The Moral Judgment of the Child* (Glencoe, IL: Free Press, 1948).

Page 41. Psychologist Lawrence Kohlberg extended and modified Piaget's theories of moral development into six stages. L. Kohlberg, "The Cognitive-developmental Approach to Socialization." In *Handbook of Socialization Theory and Research*, ed. D. A. Goslin (Chicago: Rand McNally, 1969).

Page 41. . . . "the edge girls have on moral development during the early school years gives way at puberty with the ascendance of formal logical thought in boys." C. Gilligan, *In a Different Voice: Psychological Theory and Women's Development* (Cambridge, MA: Harvard University Press, 1982).

Page 42. ". . . she finds the puzzle in the dilemma to lie in the failure of the druggist to respond to the wife." Ibid., p. 29.

Page 42. . . . gender differences in moral reasoning using Kohlberg's scales have not always been borne out and a number of theorists have tried to counter her [Gilligan's] arguments. S. Callahan, "Does Gender Make a Difference in Moral Decision Making?" *Second Opinion* 17 (October 1991): 66–77.

Page 44. "If the whole planet gets more peace, more harmony, we will get the same. Therefore each individual has a responsibility for humanity." H. H. the Dalai Lama Tenzin Gyatso, *The Opening of the Wisdom Eye* (Wheaton, IL: Quest Books, 1966), pp. v–vii.

Page 46. . . . a kind of "hundredth rat" effect. R. Sheldrake, *The Rebirth of Nature: The Greening of Science and God* (New York: Bantam Books, 1991).

Page 47. He hypothesized that the preponderance of women was due to the fact that women were more likely to write to him and describe their experiences than were men. K. Ring, *Heading Toward Omega: In Search of the Meaning of the Near-Death Experience* (New York: William Morrow, 1984), p. 29.

Page 47. Psychiatrist Frank Putnam, an expert on dissociative states, reports that the female-to-male ratio of MPD cases is approximately five to one. F. W. Putnam, *Diagnosis and Treatment of Multiple Personality Disorder* (New York: Guilford Press, 1989), p. 56.

Page 51. . . . a menstruating woman will "dim the brightness of mirrors, blunt the edge of steel and take away the polish from ivory." This quote of Pliny the Elder was cited by A. Fausto-Sterling, *Myths of Gender: Biological Theories About Women and Men*, 2d ed. (New York: Basic Books, 1992), p. 91.

Page 51. As late as the sixteenth century, medical authorities promulgated the myth that demons were produced from menstrual blood. P. Shuttle and P. Redgrove, *The Wise Wound: Myths, Realities and Meanings of Menstruation* (New York: Bantam Books, 1990).

Page 54. Do the hormonal changes that occur during the cycle affect women's perceptual abilities or emotional lives? T. Benedek and B. Rubenstein, "The Correlations Between Ovarian Activity and Psychodynamic Processes: I. The Ovulative Phase."; and "II. The Menstrual Phase," *Psychosomatic Medicine* 1 (1939): 245–70, 461–85.

Page 54. During ovulation women were content and receptive to being cared for, research that has been more recently confirmed. P. Shuttle and P. Redgrove, *The Wise Wound: Myths, Realities and Meanings of Menstruation* (New York: Bantam Books, 1990), p. 101.

Page 54. Gynecologist Christiane Northrup has expanded on the reports of Benedek and Rubenstein. . . . "Studies have shown that most women begin their menstrual periods during the dark of the moon (new moon) and begin bleeding between four and six A.M.—the darkest part of the day." C. Northrup, *Women's Bodies, Women's Wisdom* (New York: Bantam Books, 1994), p. 100.

Page 55. "If her ego is not in touch with this phase of her cycle, she often squanders her energy in increased busyness." Jungian analyst Ann Ulanov, quoted by P. Shuttle and P. Redgrove in *The Wise Wound: Myths, Realities and Meanings of Menstruation* (New York: Bantam Books, 1990), p. 119.

Page 56. Dr. Dalton has, in fact, treated some cases of PMS very successfully with natural progesterone suppositories. This fact was cited by J. R. Lee, M.D., in *What Your Doctor May Not Tell You About Menopause: The Breakthrough Book on Natural Progesterone* (New York: Warner Books, 1996), p. 64.

Page 57. One study found that fewer than 20 percent of the women who volunteered to be studied met the criteria for PMS . . . Cited by A. Fausto-Sterling, *Myths of Gender: Biological Theories About Women and Men*, 2d ed. (New York: Basic Books, 1992).

Page 58. Concerning neurophysiological correlates of negative mood premenstrually, an unexpected positive result was found. . . . "Other measures may detect enhancement of more valued right hemisphere functions premenstrually, particularly in the group of women who experience more dysphoria." M. Altemus, B. Wexler, and N. Boulis, "Neuropsychological Correlates of Menstrual Mood Changes." *Psychosomatic Medicine* 51 (1989): 329–36.

Page 58. Concerning the cycling of moods with seasons . . . But since these physiological pathways were incompletely understood fifty years ago when the study was made, the researchers considered their data "weird" and promptly scuttled it. Personal communication from L. LeShan, Ph.D.

CHAPTER FOUR
Ages 14–21: Adolescence
Snow White Falls Asleep, But Awakens to Herself

Page 61. "Fairy tales capture the essence of this phenomenon. Young women eat poisoned apples or prick their fingers with poisoned needles and fall asleep for a hundred years." M. Pipher, *Reviving Ophelia: Saving the Selves of Adolescent Girls* (New York: Ballantine Books, 1994), p. 19.

Page 61. This is not a new phenomenon. Psychologist Anne Peterson has reviewed the literature on the developmental disruption that girls experience in adolescence and traced research back to the turn of the century. A. Peterson, "Adolescent Development," *Annual Review of Psychology* 39 (1988): 583–607.

Page 64. Since the average American woman weighs 143 pounds, and fewer than one quarter of American women are taller than 5'4" . . . Data cited by K. Springen and A. Samuels, "The Body of the Beholder," *Newsweek* (24 April, 1995): 66–67.

Page 64. Boys polled at a midwestern high school found the spindly supermodel look "sickly" and "gross." Ibid.

Page 64. A study by the American Association of University Women found that 60 percent of elementary school girls were happy with themselves. By high school only 30 percent were happy. Ibid.

Page 65. Five to 15 percent of hospitalized anorexics die in treatment and only about 50 percent eventually recover. E. Uzelac, "In a Daughter's Voice," *Common Boundary* (September/October 1995): 49–53.

Page 65. In 1951 Miss Sweden was 5'7" tall and weighed 151 pounds. In 1983 Miss Sweden was 5'9" tall and weighed 109 pounds. Statistics cited by N. Wolf in *The Beauty Myth* (New York: Anchor Books, 1991), p. 182.

Page 66. It turns out that the VMN is also the site of female sexual arousal. S. LeVay, *The Sexual Brain* (Boston: MIT Press, 1993).

Page 67. ". . . The most obvious symbol is that of the full-breasted, wide-hipped, and pregnant 'Great Mother.'" C. Steiner-Adair, "The Body Politic:

Normal Female Adolescent Development and the Development of Eating Disorders." In *Making Connections: The Relational Worlds of Adolescent Girls at Emma Willard School*, ed. C. Gilligan, N. P. Lyons, and T. J. Hanmer (Cambridge, MA: Harvard University Press, 1990), pp. 162–82. Quotation from page 174.

Page 68. She has been sexually active since fifteen, like 15 percent of her female peers . . . S. S. Janus and C. L. Janus, *The Janus Report on Sexual Behavior* (New York: John F. Wiley and Sons, 1993), p. 19.

Page 73. "To seek connection with others by excluding oneself is a strategy destined to fail. . . . Is it better to respond to others and abandon themselves or to respond to themselves and abandon others? The dilemma is one of 'being a good woman, or . . . being selfish.'" C. Gilligan, "Teaching Shakespeare's Sister: Notes from the Underground of Female Adolescence." In *Making Connections: The Relational Worlds of Adolescent Girls at Emma Willard School*, ed. C. Gilligan, N. P. Lyons, and T. J. Hammer (Cambridge, MA: Harvard University Press, 1990), p. 9.

Page 73. The task of balancing depends on the development of a skill that psychologist Janet Surrey calls "relationship-authenticity" . . . J. L. Surrey, "The Self-in-Relation: A Theory of Women's Development." In *Women's Growth in Connection*, ed. J. V. Jordan, A. G. Kaplan, J. B. Miller, I. P. Stiver, and J. L. Surrey (New York: The Guilford Press, 1991).

CHAPTER FIVE
Ages 21–28: A Home of One's Own
The Psychobiology of Mating and Motherhood

Page 80. Anthropologist Helen Fisher has written a fascinating account of infatuation, marriage, and divorce in her brilliant book, *Anatomy of Love*. The outline of the discussion of infatuation was drawn from Fisher's work, although I have added several more studies on the role of pheromones. H. Fisher, *Anatomy of Love* (New York: Fawcett Columbine, 1992).

Page 81. . . . choosing men whose major histocompatibility (MHC) genes are different from their own. These data are cited in an article by S. Richardson, "The Scent of a Man." *Discover Magazine* 17 (February 1996): 26–27.

Page 85. "It was a privilege to have children, it was not a right. . . ." B. Laverdure, interviewed by S. Wall in *Wisdom's Daughters; Conversations with Women Elders of Native America* (New York: Harper Perennial, 1993), p. 130.

Page 86. Recent statistics indicate that 6.4 million American women become pregnant each year. The statistics in the next three paragraphs, including those concerning failure of contraception, were compiled by R. B. Gold and C. L. Richards, "Securing American Women's Reproductive Health." In *The*

American Woman: 1994–95, ed. C. Costello and A. J. Stone (New York: W. W. Norton, 1994).

Page 87. "In 1800, there were 7 children per woman in the United States. In 1900 there were only 3.5 and by 1940 just over 2." C. Lunardini, *What Every American Should Know About Women's History* (Holbrook, MA: Bob Adams, Inc., 1994), p. 29.

Page 88. The discussion of Margaret Sanger, Planned Parenthood, and the Comstock Law was based on the research of C. Lunardini. Ibid., p. 188.

Page 88. While abortion can be a difficult choice for women to make, almost half of all women do make it . . . S. S. Janus and C. L. Janus, *The Janus Report on Sexual Behavior* (New York: John F. Wiley and Sons, 1993), p. 220.

Page 92. . . . Agnes Simpson, a midwife who was burned at the stake in 1591 for using opium to relieve labor pains. The discussion of the role of midwives in childbirth, the prohibitions put upon them by the Roman Catholic Church, the invention of forceps, and epidemic of childbed fever was adapted from the work of A. Rich, *Of Woman Born* (New York: W. W. Norton and Company, 1986). Reissued in 1995.

Page 94. Maternal behavior begins long before birth. The biology of infatuation and the newborn is based on the discussion of B. K. Modney and G. I. Hatton. Motherhood modifies the magnocellular neuronal interrelationships in functional meaningful ways. In *Mammalian Parenting*, ed. N. A. Krasneger and R. S. Bridges (New York: Oxford University Press, 1990).

CHAPTER SIX
Ages 28–35: The Age 30 Transition
New Realities, New Plans

Page 101. The early thirties are what he calls a "structure-changing or transitional period [that] terminates the existing life structure and creates the possibility for a new one." D. J. Levinson, *The Seasons of a Woman's Life* (New York: Alfred A. Knopf, 1996), p. 25.

Page 102. Black and Hispanic women are statistically less likely to complete college, while women of Asian descent are more likely than whites to get a college degree. C. Costello and A. J. Stone, *The American Woman: 1994–95* (New York: W. W. Norton, 1994), p. 266.

Page 102. ". . . the lives of the women in our sample are therefore highly relevant to women who are now in their twenties or early thirties." G. Baruch, R. Barnett, and C. Rivers, *Lifeprints: New Patterns of Love and Work for Today's Women* (New York: Signet Books, 1983), p. 52.

Page 103. . . . "the busiest women in our study, the employed, married women with children." Ibid., p. 57.

Page 104. . . . the idea that women with children have signed up for a life of "indentured servitude." Ibid., pp. 104–106.

Page 106. . . . women trying unsuccessfully to become pregnant have stress levels, in terms of anxiety and depression, equivalent to women with cancer, HIV, and heart disease. A. D. Domar, P. Zuttermeister, and R. Friedman, "The Psychological Impact of Infertility: A Comparison with Patients with Other Medical Conditions. *Journal of Psychosomatic Obstetrics and Gynecology* 14 (1993): 45–52.

Page 106. Gynecologist Christiane Northrup ascribes unexplained infertility to five causes . . . C. Northrup, M.D., *Women's Bodies, Women's Wisdom* (New York: Bantam Books, 1994), p. 351.

Page 108. The high fat content of dairy foods also favors estrogen production . . . S. M. Lark, M.D., *Fibroid Tumors and Endometriosis: Self-Help Book* (Berkeley, CA: Celestial Arts, 1995), p. 84.

Page 108. . . . women coping with infertility are highly stressed whatever the cause; they are twice as likely to be depressed as women going to the gynecologist for routine checkups . . . A. D. Domar and H. Dreher, *Healing Mind, Healthy Woman* (New York: Henry Holt and Company, 1996), p. 223.

Page 109. . . . it has been argued that women generally score lower than men in well-being because they have primary responsibility for the children. G. Baruch, R. Barnett, and C. Rivers, *Lifeprints: New Patterns of Love and Work for Today's Women* (New York: Signet Books, 1983).

Page 109. Furthermore, the inability to prevent problems from arising is thought to make women feel vulnerable, inadequate, and incompetent . . . Ibid.

Page 112. "By their late thirties most of these career women came to understand the illusory nature of the image of Superwoman . . ." D. J. Levinson, *The Seasons of a Woman's Life* (New York: Alfred A. Knopf, 1996), p. 349.

Page 115. "What stands behind? What is not as it appears? What do I know deep in my ovaries that I wish I did not know? What of me has been killed, or lays dying?" From the story of Bluebeard. C. P. Estés, *Women Who Run with the Wolves: Myths and Stories of the Wild Woman Archetype* (New York: Ballantine Books, 1992), p. 56.

CHAPTER SEVEN
Ages 35–42: Healing and Balance
Spinning Straw into Gold

Page 120. The divorce rate has climbed from about 10 percent for couples married in 1920 . . . Statistics compiled by D. Goleman, *Emotional Intelligence* (New York: Bantam Books, 1995), p. 129.

Page 120. In trying to answer the question "Why do people divorce?" . . . H. Fisher, *Anatomy of Love* (New York: Fawcett Columbine, 1992), p. 103.

Page 121. "Hence it appears that the more children a couple bear, the less likely they are to divorce." Ibid., p. 113.

Page 122. In 1970 10.9 percent of all American households consisted of a single mother and her children. By 1991 that number had risen to 17.4 percent. Statistics compiled by C. Costello and A. J. Stone, *The American Woman: 1994–95* (New York: W. W. Norton, 1994), p. 259.

Page 122. Economically, such families are at a decided disadvantage since their average income is only about two fifths that of married couples in which both husband and wife work . . . Ibid., p. 330.

Page 123. "If we break vows for any reason other than out of obedience to a more compelling loyalty, then the situation from which we have tried to escape will simply repeat itself in another form." H. Luke, *The Way of Woman* (New York: Doubleday, 1995).

Page 125. "When a wife's face shows disgust, a near cousin of contempt . . ." J. Gottman, quoted by A. Atkisson in the review article on the Love Lab, "What Makes Love Last?" *New Age Journal* (October 1994): 74.

Page 125. Couples who are in rapport with each other actually entrain each other's autonomic nervous systems. D. Goleman, *Emotional Intelligence* (New York: Bantam Books, 1995).

Page 127. . . . even within the context of abusive or violent relationships women continue to develop valuable psychological characteristics because they "struggle to create growth-fostering interactions within the family and in other settings." J. B. Miller, *Toward a New Psychology of Women* (Boston: Beacon Press, 1976), p. xxxiii.

Page 127. One woman in four had been raped, and one woman in three had been sexually abused in childhood. A complete overview of studies and statistics concerning women and abuse, including an excellent description of "rape trauma syndrome" can be found in J. L. Herman, M.D., *Trauma and Recovery* (New York: Basic Books, 1992).

Page 129. Our conscious censors also weaken as we age, which may explain the breakthrough of traumatic memories that commonly occurs in the late thirties and forties. B. A. Van der Kolk, M.D., "The Body Keeps the Score: Memory and the Evolving Psychobiology of Posttraumatic Stress," *Harvard Review of Psychiatry* 1 (1994): 253–65.

Page 130. "Under ordinary conditions traumatized people, including rape trauma victims, battered women and abused children have a fairly good psychosocial adjustment . . ." The discussion of iconic and semantic memory and trauma is based on the research of B. A. Van der Kolk, M.D. Ibid.

Page 130. This loop has been compared to a "black hole" in the emotional circuitry that attracts every related event to itself and destroys the quality of life. R. Pittman and S. Orr, "The Black Hole of Trauma," *Biological Psychiatry* 81 (1990): 221–23.

Page 131. For example, a mouse who is locked in a box, given electric shocks, and then released will return to the box when it is stressed. J. Mitchell et al., "Habituation Under Stress: Shocked Mice Show Nonassociative Learning in a T-maze," *Behavioral Neurology and Biology* 43 (1985): 212–17.

CHAPTER EIGHT
Ages 42–49: The Midlife Metamorphosis
Authenticity, Power, and the Emergence of the Guardian

Page 142. When we feel cut off from ourselves, isolated from other people, nature, or a sense of greater power, the immune system functions at suboptimal levels. J. Borysenko and M. Borysenko, *The Power of the Mind to Heal* (Carson Beach, CA: Hay House, 1995).

Page 142. In the fascinating book *Remarkable Recovery* . . . C. Hirshberg and M. I. Barasch, *Remarkable Recovery* (New York: Riverhead Books, 1995).

Page 143. The concept of the midlife crisis, which is usually attributed to psychologist Daniel Levinson, is, he says, prone to be grossly misunderstood. D. J. Levinson, *The Seasons of a Woman's Life* (New York: Alfred A. Knopf, 1996), p. 35.

Page 145. "Their great hope was that work would provide a stronger experience of creativity, satisfaction, and social contribution . . ." D. J. Levinson. Ibid., p. 409.

Page 146. Research studies indicate that negative views of menopause also increase the number of unpleasant symptoms . . . A. D. Domar and H. Dreher, "Minding the Change: Menopause." In *Healthy Mind, Healthy Woman* (New York: Henry Holt and Company, 1996), pp. 282–310.

Page 146. "It is during perimenopause—in their forties—that women feel most estranged from their bodies. . . ." G. Sheehy, *Menopause: The Silent Passage* (New York: Pocket Books, 1993).

Page 148. The average woman completes the metamorphosis of perimenopause and emerges into the postmenopausal years when she is 48.4 years of age. *The American Woman: 1994–95*, ed. C. Costello and A. J. Stone (New York: W. W. Norton, 1995), p. 198. This statistic comes from research carried out by J. D. Forrest at the Alan Guttmacher Institute and was cited in a chapter entitled "Securing American Women's Reproductive Health," written by R. B. Gold and C. L. Richards.

Page 148. "The spirit announced to him that from then on he must sit among the women and children . . ." This is a quote from C. Jung, from *The Portable Jung*, ed. J. Campbell (New York: Penguin Books, 1976), pp. 15–16.

Page 151. Gynecologist Christiane Northrup, author of the excellent book *Women's Bodies, Women's Wisdom*, has advanced an interesting theory based on the postmenopausal rise in LH and FSH. C. Northrup, *Women's Bodies, Women's Wisdom* (New York: Bantam Books, 1994), p. 440.

Page 153. Mark Gerzon wrote a wonderful book on midlife . . . M. Gerzon, *Coming into Our Own: Understanding the Adult Metamorphosis* (New York: Delacorte Press, 1992).

Page 154. Furthermore, it is estimated that the number of women between forty-five and fifty-four will increase by one half . . . G. Sheehy, *Menopause: The Silent Passage* (New York: Pocket Books, 1993).

Page 155. "Women are essentially receptive in nature. For our first thirty-five to forty years we take the world into our being. . . ." F. Sharan, *Creative Menopause: Illuminating Women's Health and Spirituality* (Boulder, CO: Wisdome Press, 1994), p. 128.

Page 157. "It's a felt sense more than anything else. . . ." Quotation from J. Quinn, Ph.D., R.N. Personal communication as part of an interview I conducted with her for this book in March 1996.

Page 158. "Our instructions are very simple—to respect the Earth and each other, to respect life itself. . . ." Quotation from M. King, *Noble Red Man*, ed. and comp. H. Arden (Hillsboro, OR: Beyond Words Publishing, 1994), p. 11.

CHAPTER NINE
Ages 49–56: From Herbs to HRT
A Mindful Approach to Menopause

Page 160. The hypothetical Boston hospital where Julia works has taken seriously the 1993 study of Harvard physician David Eisenberg . . . D. Eisenberg et al., "Unconventional Medicine in the United States: Prevalence, Costs, and Patterns of Use," *New England Journal of Medicine* (28 January, 1993): 246–52.

Page 162. They studied thirty-three women ranging from forty-four to sixty-six years of age, whose periods had stopped for a minimum of six months, and who experienced at least five hot flashes daily. A. D. Domar and H. Dreher, *Healing Mind, Healthy Woman* (New York: Henry Holt and Company, 1996), pp. 291–92.

Page 163. The authors believe that with a larger group of women, significant reduction in hot-flash incidence would also have been observed, a result that has been reported . . . Ibid., p. 292.

Page 163. The women experienced significantly more hot flashes during lab sessions when they were subjected to a psychological stress than in a nonstress session. L. C. Swartzman, R. Edelberg, and E. Kemmann, "Impact of Stress on Objectively Recorded Menopausal Hot Flushes and on Flush Report Bias," *Health Psychology* 9 (1990): 529–45.

Page 163. British psychologist Frances Reynold of Brunel University College . . . Reported in *Mental Medicine Update: The Mind/Body Medicine Newsletter,* ed. D. Sobel, M.D., and R. Ornstein, Ph.D. 4 (1995). Both the Brunel study and the study at Guys Medical Hospital School in London, discussed in the next paragraph, were abstracts of papers presented at the annual conference of the British Psychological Association in March 1995. The papers cited in the article were those of F. Reynolds, "Suffering in Silence: Women's Experience of Menopausal Hot Flashes," and M. S. Hunter and K. L. M. Liao, "Evaluation of a Four-Session Cognitive Intervention for Menopausal Hot Flashes."

Page 165. Benson and his team found that, indeed, these monks could raise their surface temperatures . . . H. Benson et al., "Body Temperature Changes During the Practice of gTum-mo Yoga," *Nature* (1982): 295.

Page 166. "Toward the fourth month the releases increased in purity, beauty and intensity. . . ." F. Sharan, *Creative Menopause* (Boulder, CO: Wisdome Press, 1994), pp. 25–26.

Page 169. Studies indicate that 50 percent of the bone loss experienced over a woman's lifespan actually occurs *before* menopause begins . . . C. Northrup, *Women's Bodies, Women's Wisdom* (New York: Bantam Books, 1994), p. 451.

Page 171. HRT hit the mainstream in January of 1964 when *Newsweek* published an article entitled "No More Menopause . . ." This discussion is based on facts compiled by J. R. Lee, M.D., *What Your Doctor May Not Tell You About Menopause* (New York: Warner Books, 1996), pp. 189–95.

Page 172. Postmenopausal women using HRT for five or more years have a 30–40 percent greater risk of developing breast cancer than do women who do not use hormones. G. A. Colditz et al., "The Use of Estrogens and Progestins and the Risk of Breast Cancer in Post-Menopausal Women," *New England Journal of Medicine* 332 (15 June, 1995): 1589–93.

Page 173. In fact, a 1995 study in the *American Journal of Respiratory and Critical Care Medicine* reported that women on HRT . . . *Women's Health Advocate Newsletter: An Independent Voice on Women's Wellness* 2 (January 1996): 7.

Page 174. Every year 40,000 women die of breast cancer, while 250,000 die from a heart attack . . . M. J. Legato, M.D., and C. Coleman, *The Female Heart* (New York: Avon Books, 1991), p. xii.

Page 175. An article published in the *New England Journal of Medicine* in 1991 indicated that risk of death from heart disease . . . M. J. Stampfer et al., "Post-menopausal Estrogen Therapy and Cardiovascular Disease—10-year Follow-up from the Nurse's Questionnaire Study," *New England Journal of Medicine* 325 (1991): 756–62.

Page 175. In an excellent critique of this study, physician John Lee makes the point that the hormone users were also less likely . . . J. R. Lee, *What Your Doctor May Not Tell You About Menopause* (New York: Warner Books, 1996), pp. 189–95.

Page 178. Imagine that the breath is your lifeforce energy or *chi*. The *chi* breathing in this section was adapted from an exercise suggested by K. S. Cohen. Further exercises can be found in his excellent book *Strong As the Mountain, Supple As Water: The Way of Qigong* (New York: Ballantine Books, 1997).

CHAPTER TEN
Ages 56–63: The Heart of a Woman
Feminine Power and Social Action

Page 185. Sociologist Phyllis Moen and her colleagues at Cornell University conducted a thirty-year study . . . P. Moen, D. Dempster-McClain, and R. M. Williams, "Social Integration and Longevity: An Event History Analysis of Women's Roles and Resilience," *American Sociological Review* 54 (1989): 635–47; and "Successful Aging: A Life-Course Perspective on Women's Multiple Roles and Health," *American Journal of Sociology* 97 (1992): 1612–38.

Page 186. Furthermore, forty studies have found the same preponderance of depression in women in thirty different countries. D. Hales and R. E. Hales, *Caring for the Mind* (New York: Bantam Books, 1995), p. 58. The five theories on why women are more depressed than men are also taken from their excellent review on depression.

Page 186. While we can't speculate on the emotions of animals . . . M. E. P. Seligman, a psychologist at the University of Pennsylvania, has done excellent research on learned helplessness. For a review of the field, consult M. E. P. Seligman, *Helplessness: On Depression, Death and Development* (San Francisco: Freeman, 1975). An excellent book on the psychology of depression is the classic by A. T. Beck, *Depression* (New York: Hoeber, 1967).

Page 188. Imaging techniques like position emission tomography (PET scans) have been used to study changes in the brain during depression. D. Ebert and K. P. Ebermeier, "The Role of the Cingulate Gyrus in Depression: From Functional Anatomy to Neurochemistry," *Biological Psychiatry* 39 (1966): 1044–50.

Page 189. "Could the continual need to change, the continual beginnings and ends confronting women in their reproductive role have strengthened them for age? . . . " B. Friedan, *The Fountain of Age* (New York: Simon and Schuster, 1993), p. 143.

Page 190. A 1996 study by sociologist Paul Ray identified feminine values as the core of a new social movement that involves 44 million, or 24 percent of all Americans . . . P. H. Ray, "The Rise of Integral Culture," *Noetic Sciences Review* (Spring 1996): pp. 4–15. Quotation taken from p. 8.

Page 190. The Core CCs . . . are "seriously concerned with psychology, spiritual life, self-actualization, self-expression . . ." P. H. Ray. Ibid.

Page 193. Women are the fastest-growing segment of frequent moviegoers, and also rent 60 percent of the videos . . . G. Harbison, J. Ressner, and J. Savaiano, "Women of the Year," *Time* (13 November, 1995).

Page 193. A *Time* magazine article quoted Sarah Pillsbury, a Hollywood producer, on the new genre of women's films. Ibid.

Page 193. "I began to identify less with Gloria Steinem's remark at her fiftieth birthday . . ." S. Cheever, "Late Bloomer," *Living Fit* (January/February 1996).

Page 194. Nurse/researcher Janet Quinn of the University of Colorado, for example, did a study on a form of energy healing known as therapeutic touch (TT). J. F. Quinn and A. Strelkausas, "Psychophysiologic Correlates of Hands-on Healing in Practitioner and Recipients." Unpublished research report, 1987.

Page 195. Psychologist David McClelland, while a professor at Harvard, did a study concerning Mother Teresa. D. C. McClelland and C. Kirshnit, "The Effect of Motivational Arousal Through Films on Salivary Immunoglobulin-A," *Psychology and Health* 2 (1988):31–52.

Page 195. "I never look at the masses as my responsibility. I look at the individual. . . ." Mother Teresa, *Words to Love By* (Notre Dame, IN: Ave Maria Press, 1989).

Page 197. "So tractable, so peaceable are these people that I swear to Your Majesties there is not in the world a better nation. . . ." D. Brown, *Bury My Heart at Wounded Knee* (New York: Holt and Company, 1970), p. 1.

Page 197. "The world's women now converging on Beijing suddenly loom as a great force at the very moment when deadly new games of violence and greed seem to be taking over the entire world. . . ." B. Friedan, "Beyond Gender," *Newsweek* (4 December, 1995).

Page 199. "In fixing there is an inequality of expertise that can easily become a moral distance. We cannot serve at a distance . . . " R. N. Remen, "In the Service of Life," *Noetic Sciences Review* (Spring 1996): 24.

Page 199. "A nation is not conquered until the hearts of its women are on the ground . . ." M. Crow Dog with R. Erdoes, *Lakota Woman* (New York: Harper Perennial, 1990).

CHAPTER ELEVEN
Ages 63–70: Wisdom's Daughters
Creating a New Integral Culture

Page 210. In fact, the number of Americans over sixty-five has nearly tripled . . . Statistics compiled by L. Brontë and A. Pfifer, *Our Aging Society* (New York: W. W. Norton, 1986), p. 4.

Page 210. By the year 2010 the leading edge of baby boomers . . . Ibid.

Page 210. "In an aging society, it is inevitable that there will be fewer households with children. . . ." Ibid.

Page 210. In 1800, half the population was under the age of sixteen, and very few lived past sixty. Ibid.

Page 211. Eliza Pinckney was seventeen when she took over managing the family's . . . This story was told by C. Lunardini, *What Every American Should Know About Women's History* (Holbrook, MA: Bob Adams, 1994), pp. 8–9.

Page 212. "I have discovered that there is a crucial difference between society's image of old people and 'us' . . ." B. Friedan, *The Fountain of Age* (New York: Simon and Schuster, 1993), p. 31.

Page 212. She cites numerous examples of age discrimination, some of which are listed below . . . Ibid., p. 35.

Page 213. "The possibility of a new culture centers on reintegration of what has been fragmented by Modernism . . ." P. H. Ray, "The Rise of Integral Culture," *Noetic Sciences Review* (Spring 1996): 4–15. Quotation taken from p. 13.

Page 214. "Grandmother, that wonderful name, has always meant teacher in all of our society. . . ." Quotation of B. Laverdure taken from an interview by S. Wall, *Wisdom's Daughters; Conversations with Women Elders of Native America* (New York: HarperCollins, 1993), p. 132.

Page 217. "It is their system of power that is the true 'enemy of humanity' and of the earth. . . ." R. R. Ruether, *Gaia and God* (San Francisco: Harper 1992), p. 268.

Page 218. Diamond interprets her results as evidence that our brains maintain plasticity . . . M. Diamond, "Plasticity of the Aging Cerebral Cortex," *Experimental Brain Research* 5 (1982): 36–44. Supplement.

Page 218. These changes are affected by factors such as stress and sex hormones . . . M. Diamond, "Hormonal Effects on the Development of Cerebral Lateralization," *Psychoneuroimmunology* 16 (1991): 121–29.

Page 219. "There are forces at work most of us do not want to acknowledge. . . ." Quotation from an anonymous old woman reported by S. Wall, *Wisdom's Daughters; Conversations with Women Elders of Native America* (New York: HarperCollins, 1993), p. ix.

CHAPTER TWELVE
Ages 70–77: The Gifts of Change
Resiliency, Loss, and Growth

Page 224. Almost 12 percent of the total female population are widows . . . *The American Woman: 1994–95*, ed. C. Costello and A. J. Stone (New York: W. W. Norton, 1995). The statistics on longevity after widowhood in this paragraph come from this same source.

Page 224. A large body of research documents the fact that illness and death . . . A. Ciocco, "On the Mortality of Husbands and Wives," *Human Biology* 12 (1940):508–31; S. Jacob and A. Ostfeld, "An Epidemiological Review of the Mortality of Bereavement," *Psychosomatic Medicine* 39 (1977): 344–57. Also see J. J. Lynch, *The Broken Heart: The Medical Consequences of Loneliness* (New York: Basic Books, 1977).

Page 224. A large number of studies have shown that social connectedness is an important buffer against all kinds of stress and loss . . . L. F. Berkman and S. L. Syme, "Social Networks, Host Resistance and Mortality: A Nine-Year Follow-up Study of Alameda County Residents," *American Journal of Epidemiology* 109 (1979):186–224.

Page 224. Psychologist Janice Kiecolt-Glaser and her husband, immunologist Ronald Glaser, from Ohio State Medical School found that lonely people . . . For review of this and other of their work, see J. K. Kiecolt-Glaser and R. Glaser, "Psychosocial Moderators of Immune Function," *Annals of Behavioral Medicine* 9 (1987): 16–20.

Page 225. Even the simple act of confessing one's trauma to a shower curtain . . . This and other studies on confession and healing are discussed in J. W. Pennebaker, "Confession, Inhibition and Disease," *Advances in Experimental Social Psychology* 22 (1989): 212–44. Immunological benefits of confession are discussed in J. W. Pennebaker, J. K. Kiecolt-Glaser, and R. Glaser, "Disclosure of Traumas and Immune Function: Health Implications for Psychotherapy," *Journal of Consulting and Clinical Psychology* 56 (1988): 239–45.

Page 225. Psychologist Martin Seligman of the University of Pennsylvania found that pessimistic people, who tend to feel helpless, often blame themselves . . . M. E. P. Seligman, *Learned Optimism* (New York: Alfred A. Knopf, 1991), chap. 10.

Page 226. Psychologist Suzanne Ouellette, of the City College of New York, has studied optimistic, resilient people . . . S. O. Kobasa, "Stressful Life Events, Personality and Health: An Inquiry into Hardiness," *Journal of Personality and Social Psychology* 37 (1979): 1–11. (She changed her name from Kobasa to Ouellette, so earlier articles can be found under her previous name.)

Page 226. When rats are subjected to shock, for example, those animals who consistently hear a buzzer . . . J. M. Weiss, "Psychological Factors in Stress and Disease," *Scientific American* (June 1972). For the effects of helplessness on stress and tumor growth, see M. A. Visintainer, J. R. Volpicelli, and M. E. P. Seligman, "Tumor Rejection in Rats after Inescapable or Escapable Shock," *Science* 216 (1982): 437–39.

Page 228. In fact, when pruning fails to occur in the young brain, there is an increased instance of mental retardation . . . J. Hooper and D. Teresi, *The 3-Pound Universe* (New York: Macmillan Publishing Company, 1986); and M. L. Shulz, M.D., Ph.D,. personal communication.

Page 229. "I have no romantic feelings about age. Either you are interesting at any age or you are not." This quote from Katharine Hepburn was cited by G. Dianda and B. Hoffmayer in *Older and Wiser* (New York: Ballantine Books, 1995), p. 125.

Page 229. Harvard psychologist Ellen Langer and her Yale colleague Judith Rodin believe that people who stay engaged with life . . . Langer's large body of research is summarized in her excellent book *Mindfulness* (Reading, MA: Addison Wesley, 1989).

Page 230. DHEA is the most common and abundant of the steroid hormones . . . For a complete review of the structure, function, and possible clinical utility of DHEA, see C. N. Shealy, M.D., Ph.D., *DHEA: The Youth and Health Hormone* (New Canaan, CT: Keats Publishing, Inc., 1996).

Page 231. Dr. John Lee, a physician whose interest in the use of natural progesterone to relieve PMS and menopausal symptoms . . . J. R. Lee, *What Your Doctor May Not Tell You About Menopause* (New York: Warner Books, 1996), p. 141.

Page 231. Physician and researcher Dean Ornish, author of *Dr. Ornish's Program for Reversing Coronary Artery Disease*, has published numerous articles . . . see D. M. Ornish et al., "Can Lifestyle Changes Reverse Coronary Atherosclerosis? The Lifestyle Heart Trial," *Lancet* 336 (1990):129–33.

Page 231. Once again, social support shows up as an important factor both in the genesis and treatment of cardiovascular disease. For a thorough review of the effects of stress, environment, social support, and personality factors in heart disease, see the proceedings of a conference on Behavioral Medicine and Cardiovascular Disease, J. T. Shepherd and S. M. Weiss.

Page 233. Psychologist Janice Kiecolt-Glaser and her husband, immunologist Ronald Glaser, studied elderly people in nursing homes. J. Kiecolt-Glaser et al., "Psychosocial Enhancement of Immunocompetence in a Geriatric Population," *Health Psychology* 4 (1985): 25–41.

Page 234. A 1995 study in the prestigious *Journal of the American Medical Association* documented serious shortcomings in communication between seriously ill hospitalized patients and their physicians. "The SUPPORT Principal Investigators, A Controlled Trial to Improve Care for Seriously Ill Hospitalized Patients." *Journal of the American Medical Association* 274 (1995):1591–97.

Page 239. Seventy percent of women are still healthy in their seventies . . . Statistics cited in C. Costello and A. J. Stone, *The American Woman: 1994–95* (New York: W. W. Norton, 1994), p. 229.

CHAPTER THIRTEEN
Ages 77–84 and Beyond: Recapitulating Our Lives
Generativity, Retrospection, and Transcendence

Page 240. At eighty Julia is unmarried like 75 percent of the women in her age bracket. The statistics in the first two paragraphs are drawn from C. Costello and A. J. Stone, *The American Woman: 1994–95* (New York: W. W. Norton, 1994), pp. 231–32.

Page 241. "I remember the old woman who cleaned the floor in my place in Gargenville. . . ." This quotation from N. Boulanger came from D. G. Campbell, *Master Teacher: Nadia Boulanger* (Washington, DC: The Pastoral Press, 1984), p. 64.

Page 242. This story concerns two pampered elders, eighty and seventy-five, who have allowed themselves to be coddled by their tribe . . . This story was told by V. Wallis in *Two Old Women: An Alaska Legend of Betrayal, Courage and Survival* (New York: Harper Perennial, 1993).

Page 248. Neuroscientist Marcel Mesulam, of Northwestern University in Chicago, is intrigued by the fact that blood clots and small strokes preferentially affect the short-term memory of elders . . . Personal communication, M. L. Schulz, M.D., Ph.D.

Page 249. "In the beginning were the Instructions. We were to have compassion for one another . . ." This quote from V. Downey was cited by S. Wall in *Wisdom's Daughters; Conversations with Women Elders of Native America* (New York: Harper Perennial, 1994), p. 2.

Page 251. "Every life is a circle. And within every life are smaller circles. . . ." This quote from B. M. Adams was cited by N. S. Hill in *Words of Power: Voices from Indian America* (Golden, CO: Fulcrum Publishing, 1994), p. 38.

INDEX